Culpeper's
Complete
Astrology

∿ The **∿**

LOST ART
of ASTROLOGICAL
MEDICINE

Nicholas Culpeper

introduction by Judith Hill

foreword by Alice Sparkly Kat

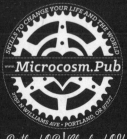

Portland, OR | Cleveland, OH

Culpeper's Complete Astrology: The Lost Art of Astrological Medicine

This edition © Microcosm Publishing, 2023

This edition first published October 17, 2023

Book design by Joe Biel

Cover by Lindsey Cleworth

Edited by Lex Orgera

ISBN 9781648413056

This is Microcosm #814

Library of Congress Control Number: 2023028071

MICROCOSM · PUBLISHING

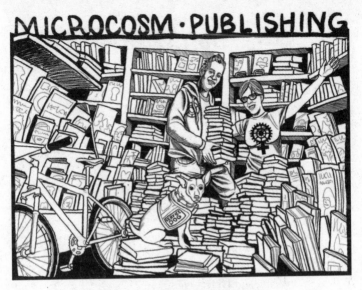

About the Publisher

MICROCOSM PUBLISHING is Portland's most diversified publishing house and distributor, with a focus on the colorful, authentic, and empowering. Our books and zines have put your power in your hands since 1996, equipping readers to make positive changes in their lives and in the world around them. Microcosm emphasizes skill-building, showing hidden histories, and fostering creativity through challenging conventional publishing wisdom with books and bookettes about DIY skills, food, bicycling, gender, self-care, and social justice. What was once a distro and record label started by Joe Biel in a drafty bedroom was determined to be *Publishers Weekly*'s fastest-growing publisher of 2022 and #3 in 2023, and is now among the oldest independent publishing houses in Portland, OR, and Cleveland, OH. We are a politically moderate, centrist publisher in a world that has inched to the right for the past 80 years.

Contents

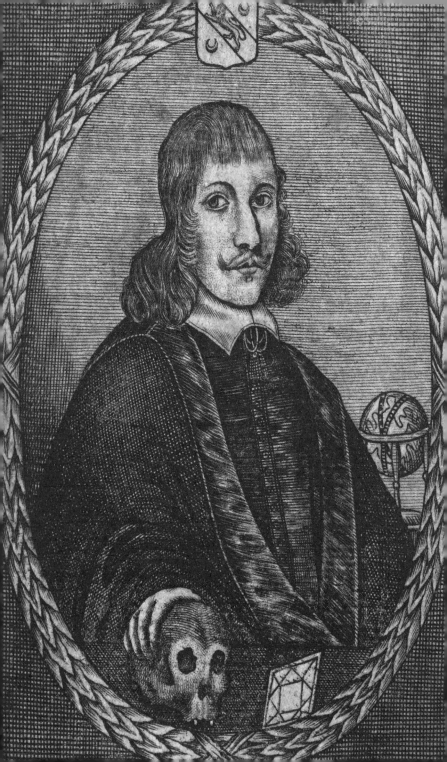

Foreword

Alice Sparkly Kat

More than Medicine

There are many reasons why someone might go to an astrologer when preparing for something like, say, a surgery.

Surgeries are physical. They usually happen behind closed doors with medical professionals we trust to know what they are doing. We usually think of them happening with blades on bodies, the site of surgery contained to the body being cut.

Surgeries are also life events. They affect an entire kinship network. One person's surgery can affect a whole community. Surgeries interrupt work, which means that they can impact a workplace. They can impact all of the people you serve if your work involves working with people. People who undergo surgery require care. Surgeries can expose needs and gaps in relationships, in family systems, in entire communities. They can destabilize existing dynamics, and they can create new opportunities for connection. They can create new opportunities for rejection. Surgeries can change someone's life and not just in the ways that they were expecting. The impact of a surgery can sometimes be felt long after the event is over, not just in the way that the cells grow around what was removed but through changes in how people move together, realized long after a new need was made clear. Surgeries cut socially as well as physically.

People might be interested in astrological consultation before they go into surgery but also years after a surgery has already happened.

I bring this up not because Nicholas Culpeper goes into surgeries so much in his book *An Astrological Judgment of Diseases from the Decumbiture of the Sick* but as an example of why people might seek astrological metaphor when healing in general, from chicken pox or a broken leg or when trying to understand long-term chronic pain.

An astrologer can provide a helpful framework for disease, comfort in the face of scary circumstances, and sometimes even a sense of humor.

Culpeper certainly had a sense of humor. In *Astrological Judgment of Diseases*, he shows you how to distinguish between an illness of the body and instances where "some idle Priest has scar'd the poor creature out of his wits." I imagine that he was quite funny with the people he worked with too.

He was also considered to be a bit of a radical in his day, choosing to publish self-help manuals for poor people with recipes for cheap herbal cures instead of expensive concoctions. He wrote in English instead of Latin so that more people could read what he had to say. Culpeper was a noble himself, but he saw medicine as overly gatekept and only sold cheap books or remedies. He thought that the high price of medicine itself was a disease. Working with as many as forty people per day, Culpeper helped the working poor with everything from lice and losses of appetite to relief of gas.

A Tale of Mugwort

One of the plants that Culpeper worked with was mugwort. Mugwort, in small quantities, has been used to ease menstrual pain. In larger quantities, mugwort has been used to either induce labor or for abortion purposes. Mugwort can be ingested, infused as tea, or rolled up in some papers and smoked. People make cakes, pancakes, or buns using mugwort (simply steam it coated with wheat flour!). Ingesting mugwort can induce vivid dreams or even lucid dreams. For some people, mugwort can produce hallucinations.

The first time I encountered mugwort was with my family in Henan, China. We were never really good at keeping track of dates, and one morning we realized that it was Zongzi Day only when a neighbor brought us a huge bushel of mugwort. In Henan, it's customary to hang mugwort, called aicao, on your door on Zongzi Day for protection. (Zongzi Day is actually the Dragon Boat Festival, but because we eat a food called zongzi during the festival, my family has always called it Zongzi Day—to the point where no one remembers the real name when pressed!). We hung the aicao on the front door, relieved that someone else remembered for us.

Mugwort grows thick in parking lots, along chain link fences, and in gutters where I live in the US. If you're not careful, mugwort will quickly overtake a park field. It was introduced to the continent in the sixteenth century by Jesuit missionaries.

Culpeper writes in his *Complete Herbal* that mugwort is ruled by Venus. This is why mugwort aids with birth and with menstruation. It is also why mugwort helps with neck and throat pain when mixed with oil because Taurus describes the throat in astrology and Venus rules Taurus. It is helpful to know that mugwort is ruled by Venus because Venus describes mugwort through a world of biological experiences, body parts, and cycles.

Sympathy as Medicine

Astrological Judgment of Diseases is a historical document. In it, Culpeper describes disease. He notes things like whether a fever is short or long, whether a sweat is hot or cold, and investigates whether a disease is caused by antipathy or sympathy. When Culpeper does not know something, he says so. When he shares something that he has learned but not experienced, he writes that he has not yet consulted Dr. Experience. In one section, Culpeper notes that cases where the lord of the sixth house and the lord of the eighth house are in harmonious aspect tend to turn out well when he thinks that the reverse should be true. He believed that when disease and death are in harmony, this should be an ominous sign—and he informs the reader that he does not always know why things happen the way they do.

The way that Culpeper describes disease is intimate, not institutional. He describes a sick young woman who had Venus in Sagittarius. He notes that she is unhappy in her marriage, with a husband who is not well matched to her, and that her physician had bad eyesight. He notes the position of the Moon throughout all three of the crises she underwent, suggesting that he was close by her side as she suffered. Culpeper is primarily concerned with how the astrological signatures speak to the question of whether she will live or die. He seems completely uninterested in the classification of the woman's disease. He seems much more concerned with her, her inner life, and whether she will live or die.

Why might someone seek a description of their illness as a retrograde motion of Venus or an application of the Moon to Saturn? Why might people seek metaphorical companionship when we suffer?

It might be because there is truth in metaphor. Astrology works in mysterious ways. We might also seek astrological companionship in sickness for the same reasons that we are more interested in a plant's symbolism, smell, and taste than its chemistry. Why we might seek counsel over a surgery that occurred years in the past, why we look to the sky for answers to questions of life or death—there is truth in metaphor because there is memory in metaphor.

Once, I had a client come to me. One of the things that they asked to discuss during our consultation together was their vision and practice of community. During that session, the client told me a story about a Mars opposition. It just so happened that they had a surgery during that Mars opposition some time before our session. What does Mars have to do with community? What do surgeries have to do with community? Astrological sympathy is the study of how meanings mirror and link to other meanings. My client told me a story about how surgery, and Mars along with it, interrupted their community relationships necessarily so that they could find more honesty. This is Mars, working through sympathy, in their life.

Sometimes, the classification of an illness or condition of suffering gives us the language we need to speak about our lives. Sometimes, the classification of our experiences also teaches us how to suffer legibly. Sometimes, we need more than classification. We need magical thinking. We need to know, for instance, that mugwort is associated with Venus, that it has a relationship to menstruation, that it works through dreams, and we find what it looks and smells like through story. We need to know that Mars works through both surgeries and conflicts, that Venus was in retrograde during the time of our illness, and that we survived a Moon-Saturn conjunction.

We are often more concerned about what plants we can eat and which ones we cannot than about the scientific classification of plants, for the same reasons that we are more concerned about questions of life and death than the classification of disease. *Astrological Judgment of Diseases* narrates illness both metaphorically and magically and gives us another language to draw from.

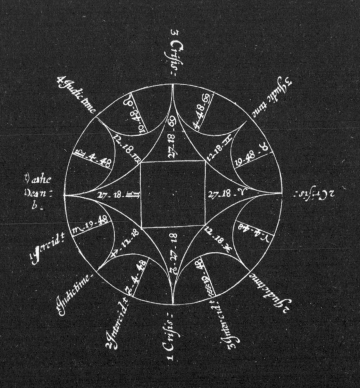

~Introduction~

Judith Hill

Medical Astrology, the use of astrological charts for medical purposes, flourished as a comprehensive medical system during Nicholas Culpeper's lifetime. Culpeper wrote his seminal *An Astrological Judgment of Diseases from the Decumbiture of the Sick* to assist students of astrological medicine in the art of interpreting the decumbiture chart and its companion chart, the Crucial Circle.[1]

Decumbiture comes from the Latin *decumbo*, meaning "to fall or lie down." A decumbiture, then, is a horoscope calculated for the time the patient took to the bed. Culpeper didn't invent the technique; decumbiture had been around from at least the time of its first known BCE mentions in works by Petosiris and Hermes.

The decumbiture chart Culpeper espoused was used to discern disease cause, predict crises, give prognoses, and select remedies appropriate to specific patients. However, from the physician's point of view, there was a further overarching concern for casting decumbitures, being, "Will my patient die?" A dead patient sullied one's reputation. The average seventeenth-century English lifespan was thirty-five so this was a legitimate concern. Unsanitary conditions, recurrent plagues, wars, high infant mortality, plus the chronically "binding" London diets of largely beer, meats, dairy products, breads, and grains (plus the occasional leek, carrot, or cabbage), that all contributed to

---

1 Curiously, Culpeper never actually states the distinct term for this important and popular adjunct technique used to discern crisis dates and prognoses. Rather than using the term Crucial Circle, he discusses how to find the "critical and judicial days" and then details the precise technique. The use of the term Crucial Circle for this method is found in contemporary Joseph Blagrave's guidebook *Blagrave's Astrological Practice of Physick*.

frequent patient loss. (Era physician Joseph Blagrave cites constipation as a significant cause of insanity! Without antibiotics, an infected tooth might carry you away!) Culpeper and his colleagues might very well decline a patient whose decumbiture foretold approaching fatality. Another good reason for decumbiture's popularity during this time was strictly legal. Natal, or "genethliacal," astrology was prohibited for general use; whereas, both natal charts used for medical purposes and decumbitures, which were already used for purely medical purposes, were permissible. Those who dared cast natal charts for reasons other than medical practice might well find themselves in the Tower of London (as befell John Dee in 1555 for casting the horoscopes of Queen Anne and Princess Elizabeth).

Culpeper was both a practitioner and defender of this ancient medical technology. He and his colleagues created what might well be termed the "Great British Golden Age" of Medical Astrology and Astrological Herbalism. As both master herbalist and astrologer, the generous Culpeper was beloved amongst the common folk who disdained the institutional doctors who sauntered about the realm in elegant footwear spewing cryptic Latin while exacting large fees from their poor and illiterate patients. In return, the institutional doctors hated Culpeper.

English Astrological Herbalism and the art of decumbiture flourished at a time when newly industrializing London was swarming with rural emigres. The British countryside was fast depopulating. Shorn of their herb gardens and "cunning folk," London's poor turned to those who could offer them affordable diagnosis and familiar herbs. Culpeper was born to the task.

Seventeenth-century medical practice stood delicately poised between King Henry's 1542 protective Herbalist's Charter, the witchcraft trials of the mid-1620s, and the shrill hostility of London's Royal College of Physicians. Yet, for a few remarkable decades, anatomical advances and scientific inquiry existed commodiously alongside the old knowledge of planets, elves, and unseen forces. Culpeper and his fellow "people's" herbalists were uneasily shielded from the livid persecutions of the university physicians, the Church, and the King—unless, of course, their profits were threatened.

Medical Astrology, known at the time as "astrologo-physic" enjoyed a renewed protected status as well. Pope John III's Tridentine Council ruled in 1563 that "natural" astrology was, in fact, legal. Natural astrology was essential to weather prediction, planting, plague alerts, political concerns, predicting the success of the King's armies, and the healing craft. Culpeper's oft-reiterated quote echoed the sentiments of his time toward the practical utility of the art:

> "A physician without astrology is like a pudding without fat."

His sentiment is echoed in this laudatory poem by Lancelot Coelson in his foreword to a contemporaneous text on this topic by London's rival "master of the decumbiture," Richard Saunders:

> "...For who without Astrology would know,
>
> The Art of Healing, does but blindfold go,
>
> By dull conjectures they are wandering led
>
> Into a labyrinth without a thread..."

These pithy poetics, while typical of astrologo-physicians, were not merely entertaining but intended to defend an art facing manifold threats. Despite multivarious opposition (that would effectively derail the system by 1700), the knowledge of planetary-physical effects was considered so medically essential that license-aspiring medical students needed to pass their astrological exams until 1666.

Culpeper was not the sole Renaissance writer to publish a detailed tutorial on decumbiture, though it was tenuously dangerous to publish on the topic. William Lilly's chapter on health questions appears in his famous tome, *Christian Astrology* (1647). Then, Culpeper's 1651 text *An Astrological Judgment of Diseases from the Decumbiture of the Sick*, exclusive to decumbiture and Crucial Circle technique, was followed by Joseph Blagrave's remarkable *Blagrave's Astrological Practice of Physic*, first published in 1671 and Richard Saunders' 1677 *The Astrological Judgment and Practice of Physic: Deducted from the Position of the Heavens at the Decumbiture of the Sick Person*. Lilly, Culpeper, Blagrave, and Saunders offer the avid student several variations of technique. Culpeper's method, detailed in this present book, is perhaps the most widely used today.

More on Charts

The radix (birth chart) provides the physician a far more holistic knowledge of the patient's innate patterns than does a decumbiture. The birth chart can assess multiple levels of being (mental, emotional, physical) and describe the permanently embedded energetic template informing the body. Natal charts, and transits acting upon them, were definitely utilized in Culpeper's time for medical purposes, and large collections exist. However, for practical purposes because exact birthdays and times were hard to come by other than with royalty, decumbiture was the prevalent period technique.

Decumbiture as part of "natural" astrology enjoyed protected status. The 1563 Tridentine Council legislated astrological genres into two distinct camps: "Natural" (legal) and "Judicial" (prohibited). "Natural" included astrology's medical, meteorological, and agricultural branches; whereas, "Judicial" astrology concerned predictions—hence interfering with God's will. The exclusive use of decumbiture charts for medical purposes rendered them legally safe. Conversely, the casting of natal (birth) charts ran the practitioner a terrible risk of arrest, being as these were equally applicable to both medical (legal), and "judicial" purposes (prohibited).

Curiously, decumbiture's partial use as a prognostic tool for medical outcome was permitted!

God had no problem whatsoever with the Culpeper's work, but the Royal College of Physicians sure did!

Supposedly, astrologo-physicians could practice freely without fear of prosecution, as long as they avoided all semblance of witchcraft. (The Witchcraft Act was passed in 1563, the same year that Medical Astrology was deemed legal). Despite such official protections, Culpeper's enemies at the Royal College of Physicians were incensed by his "people's" approach. He broke the rules by writing instructive books in plain English, charging affordable fees, and founding an apothecary stocked with affordable, local herbs. They waged a campaign of defamation against his work and managed twice to scramble up charges of witchcraft, a potentially mortal charge. It was a dangerous time for any healer working outside of the Royal College's approval! It was into this strained atmosphere that Culpeper published his three seminal works: In 1652 he completed the *The English Physician*, and only one year following, an expansion of this initial text entitled *The Complete Herbal* (1653). Culpeper empirically tested the astrological-herbal system, finding it sound. Here, in the habit of his times, he lauds his own text:

> *"The English Physician: or an Astrologo-Physical Discourse of the Vulgar Herbs of this Nation.* Being a Complete Method of Physic, whereby a man may preserve his Body in Health, or cure himself, being sick, for three pence charge, with such things only as grow in England, they being most fit for English Bodies."

Our present text initiates this trilogy: *An Astrological Judgment of Diseases from the Decumbiture of the Sick* (1651). Three great works in three years! It is apparent that Culpeper was hurriedly preserving this complete Western medical system as it dangled on the veritable knife's edge of threatened extinction.

The British Golden Age of Medical Astrology

What made the British "Golden Age of Medical Astrology" uniquely exciting in the history of astrological medicine?

In a curious twist of fate, Culpeper plus at least eight influential, fellow astrologo-physicians were all born within twenty-five years of each other within a close proximity to the environs of London, where their lives converged. Pertinently, these men were born either during the later life of, or within nineteen years following the death of the remarkable genius, astrologo-physician, mathematician, inventor, and magus, John Dee (1527-1608). As an astrological herbalist and creator of the arguably largest library in the sixteenth century world—over three thousand rare volumes—Dee kept fascinating case notes on ailments and herbal cures. Culpeper's colleagues followed in Dee's inspired footsteps, creating more libraries. For example, Culpeper's contemporary and guild fellow Elias Ashmole amassed a magnificent library of over 200 volumes, housed at Lambeth, South London. Dee's thirst for knowledge influenced the upcoming generation of British health practitioners, including young Nicholas Culpeper, born but eight years following Dee's mysterious death.

The serendipitous mix of the eight-plus London personalities immediately succeeding Dee could be likened to Florence's artistic Renaissance. Today's astrologers still revere John Dee, Simon Foreman, Elias Ashmole, Joseph Blagrave, William Lilly ("The English Merlin"), John Gadbury, Richard Saunders ("The English Apollo"), Richard Napier, and, of course, Nicholas Culpeper. And they all wrote! Some recorded medical case studies, others wrote "how to" guides on various astrological topics inclusive of astrological medicine, while still others amassed research collections of horoscopes.

Most were voluminous writers, in fact. Saunders published his compendium of decumbiture cases twenty-five years following Culpeper's *Judgment*. Significant medical case notes, replete with horoscopes and crudely "modern" intake notes were also produced by Napier, Ashmole, Blagrave, and the maverick physician Foreman. The infamous Foreman even diaried his sexual exploits alongside his medical cases with the same brilliant clarity!

The 1453 invention of the printing press made possible the rapid dissemination of their astrological ideas and discoveries to the public. No longer was astrological expertise confined to the intellectual elite. Astrological almanacs were all the rage among the seventeenth-century English populace—one infamous almanac was penned by Culpeper's first astrological tutor and fellow "people's physician," William Lilly (today remembered more for his having predicted the Great Fire of London).

These nine leading astrologo-medical thinkers were as stimulated by the budding Enlightenment as were any other academic fellowship. Following suit with other sciences, astrologers began to found societies, craft libraries, document their cases, write more detailed books than ever seen before, and question tradition. We find Culpeper's contemporary Richard Saunders very much of this spirit in his questioning of the rigid rules applied to decumbiture! In the spirit of science, astrologo-physicians were an inventive lot, thinking for themselves. This only furthered the ire of their enemies. Culpeper, Lilly, Ashmole, and others were determined to raise the stature and professionality of their mutual field. It was time to come on par with other professional guilds. The result was "The London Society of Astrologers," founded in 1647, boasting about forty members.

The society met twice yearly at Gresham College, Bishopsgate and also delighted in "Astrologer's Feasts" held at various pubs where they enjoyed an opening sermon, shared instruments, furthered the state of their art, and feasted. We can envision Culpeper and Lilly sharing an Englishman's beef and beer whilst delighting in a fellow's presentation on the practical points of decumbiture!

Precisely as astrological medicine achieved its finest hour, the bells of cultural banishment chimed loudly. The threatened university physicians joined ideological forces with the new astronomers and their telescopes. After all, the secret was out that the earth was no longer at the center of the universe, and thus astrology must be errant. Furthermore, because Galen had gotten the anatomy wrong, his entire medical system was invalidated. Or, so chanted his excoriators.

One could proffer that it was this very gathering of Western resistance to astrological thought that partially force-fed the finest moment of astrologo-physic. Astrology has always known what Saunders called its "carping critics," but resistance from both the self-appointed newly enlightened physicians and scientists was now met by a vigorous counter thrust, unnecessary within previous astrology-safe cultures.

During this time, a torrent of collective works by Culpeper, Blagrave, Lilly, Saunders, Foreman, Ashmole, Gadbury, et al., gushed forth precisely as astrological medicine was banned from the universities (1666) and Galenism was in tatters (a process begun eighty some years previous with new anatomical and astronomical discoveries, including Harvey's discoveries about human circulation in 1583).

The astrological-herbal medical system Culpeper espoused was every bit as complex and venerable as Traditional Chinese Medicine, or India's Ayurvedic medicine. Western Astrological Herbalism was a triune system: consisting of astrology, herbs, and patient examination (pulse, tongue, pallor, urine, feces, humor balance, and innate temperament.) However, the crown jewel of the system was astrology. The natal chart, transits, decumbiture, the Crucial Circle, plus current transits, provided the practitioner a kind of cosmic microscope for viewing the energetic template behind physical form, pathology, and the universal tides. Furthermore, natal charts, decumbitures, and Crucial Circle charts were used to determine the cause, length, and cure of disease.

Culpeper and his colleagues recognized a far wider palette of disease origins than do today's physicians. First, Culpeper would discern if the disease was "natural" or "supernatural." This was determined through the decumbiture chart. Should the time of onset be unknown, he would calculate the chart from the first moment of patient contact, or the time their urine was presented for analysis. Hence, the unfortunate epithet attached to many of England's astrological physicians: "piss prophets."

Etiologies considered included: astrological causation, bad food, foul air, weather disturbance of "humors," constipation, emotional shock, parental inheritance, childbirth (opening of the womb), elf-shot, fairy revenge, bewitchment, spirit possession, and of supreme importance: "of God." With no concept of reincarnation, genetics, or karma, this last designation sufficed for "born that way." Astrological influences were viewed as obvious sources of disease in their own right, while simultaneously regarded as a primary means for discerning all other etiologies!

Culpeper Today

Today, most know little, if anything, about the ancient and effective triune medical system. Curiously (and sadly), we have, in fact, no usefully descriptive modern word for it! This oversight was due in part to its fanatically vigorous suppression at the close of the seventeenth century, in what might be termed the Great Abandonment. Should Culpeper have published his *Astrological Judgment of Diseases* together in one volume with his *Complete Herbal*, perhaps this system as an entirety would not have so quickly occluded. Regretfully, he did not, and few today realize how connected these two works actually are! Together, both *The Complete Herbal* and

An Astrological Judgment of Diseases from the Decumbiture of the Sick comprise two legs of the three-legged stool of astrologo-physic. (The third leg being patient examination).

Despite the suppression suffered, the astrological techniques of this ancient medical system lived on, albeit underground. Throughout the Great Abandonment of the eighteenth century, until our present day, one always finds some renegade doctor, somewhere, utilizing these same venerable techniques.

The last ten years have witnessed a springtime of interest in Western Astrological-Herbal medicine and Medical Astrology. "Modern" medical astrology began in the early twentieth century and continues through the present day. The early modern medical astrologers preferred use of the natal chart and transits to the decumbiture method. Nativities are readily available now and should be obtained when possible!

However, provided one obtains an exact onset time, decumbiture performs well as a useful "test tube of time," allowing the practitioner a close-up, second opinion of a known medical event.

Decumbiture remains useful to the modern practitioner when:

a)   it is illegal or embarrassing to request birth data;

b)   birth data cannot be readily obtained;

c)   there is no time available to calculate and study the full natal chart.

Occasional medical practitioners utilize natal charts, transits, decumbitures, "consulting charts," Crucial Circles, and astrological herbalism in their twenty-first-century practices. Today, small clinics exist whose practitioners set charts for the time of each client consult, exactly as Culpeper might have. A generation of "Post-Moderns" has now arrived, busily combining decumbiture with acupuncture, sound healing, homeopathy, and more.

We can thank Culpeper and his comrades for preserving an ancient medical technology still viable today. Should medical astrology have nothing to offer or add to modern clinical medicine, then its study would be exclusively academic. However, it is quite the reverse! Clinical medicine cannot yet see into the unseen energies behind innate temperament and disease or discern the timing for onset of illness or mortal threat. Best times for hospital release cannot be properly known without a guide into the unseen forces at play upon the body. Neither can safest surgery dates be accurately discerned. Medical Astrology can identify the seat of disease, provide accurate prognosis, and assist the selection of best remedies. Or so thought Culpeper and countless others down the centuries who have empirically tested the system and found it sound.

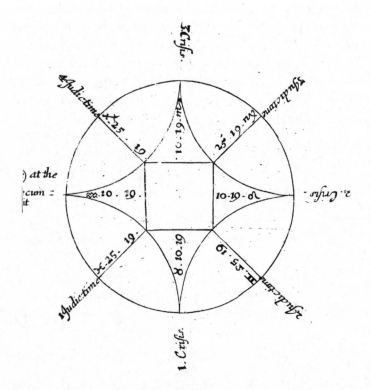

3. Crisis.

3 Judicatiun̄.

4 Judicatiun̄.

1. Crisis.

2 Judicatiun̄.

2. Crisis.

1. Crisis.

) at the
cum =
it

Publisher's Note

Nicholas Culpeper's *Semeiotica Uranica, or, An Astrological Judgment of Diseases from the Decumbiture of the Sick* was originally published in 1651. In addition to highlighting Culpeper's snarky wit and his famous consultations with Dr. Reason and Dr. Experience, *Astrological Judgment of Diseases* is a synthesis (and often a direct translation) of the works of three important thinkers: Hippocrates (often by way of the Roman-Greek physician Galen), Abraham Ibn Ezra, and Noël Duret. While many are familiar with Hippocrates as the ancient Greek father of medicine, Ibn Ezra and Duret are less well known, and Culpeper's variant spellings of their names called for short footnotes introducing them to readers.

We used the 1651 edition provided by the Text Creation Partnership at the University of Michigan Library (a partnership between the University of Michigan Library, Bodleian Libraries at the University of Oxford, ProQuest, and the Council on Library and Information Resources). The corresponding illustrations are from the 1671 edition of the scanned manuscript at the Internet Archive. The 1651 edition and later editions published after Culpeper's death in 1654 vary quite a bit; for instance, later editions include added chapters and sections, such as a chapter with a table of logarithms to help calculate a crisis, as well as a section titled "Hermes Trismegistus: Upon the First Decumbiture of the Sick." We didn't include any sections that were not in the 1651 text.

Culpeper's astrological, herbal, and medical texts were purposely accessible to a wide audience (at least folks who could read English) during a time when medical knowledge was written in Latin and closely guarded by the elite. In the spirit of accessibility to a modern audience, and for the purposes of maximum readability, we have standardized and updated some of Culpeper's spellings, corrected confusing grammar, and added clarifying punctuation. We attempted to use a light hand, generally leaving Culpeper's sentence constructions and creative capitalizations intact because, while a little odd to the modern eye, they contribute to the unique voice and flavor of the text.

A note on standardization in the seventeenth century: Culpeper's own signature at the end of the text is spelled with two p's—Culpepper—and we've left that as is.

Semeiotica Uranica. Or an Astrological Judgment of Diseases from the Decumbiture of the Sick

1. From Aven Ezra by way of Introduction.

2. From Noel Duret by way of Direction.

Wherein is laid down,

The way and manner of finding out the Cause, Change, and End of a Disease. Also whether the Sick be likely to live or die, and the Time when Recovery or Death is to be expected.

To which is added The Signs of Life or Death by the body of the Sick Party according to the judgment of Hippocrates.

By NICHOLAS CULPEPER Gent. Student in Physic and Astrology.

PERSIUS.

Disce, sed ira cadat naso, rugosa (que) sanna.

London, Printed for Nathaniel Brookes at the Golden Angel on Cornhill, near the Exchange. 1651.

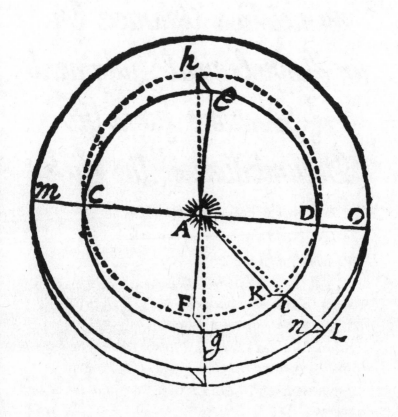

dedication

To the astrologers of England,
Nicholas Culpeper wishes peace
and prosperity in this world, and
eternal beatitude in that which is to come.

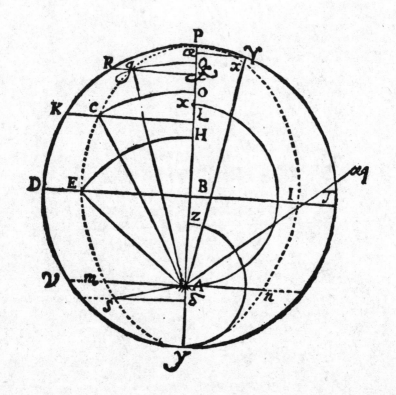

note to readers 1

Dear Souls,

To you all, and to you especially that heard these Lectures, do I dedicate them, and present them to you, not to look upon only (for then I had as good have sent you a picture, and as much it would have pleased your eye). Man was made not only for Speculation, but also for Practice; Speculation brings only pleasure to a man's self; it's Practice which benefits others; And I hope I need not tell you that Man was not born for himself alone. These Rules will serve (if heedfully observed by the eye of Reason) to balance your judgment in sailing through the Prognostical part of the Physic, that so you may steer your course by the Card of Truth, and not float unsettled upon the waves of Error, Ignorance or Opinion. To you (rather than to any that I know) belongs the practice of Physic; and that Practice may be perfect, judgment ought to be sound; and to make judgment sound is required an exquisite knowledge. Judgment is perfected by knowledge, knowledge by experience: whence it appears, that the more communicative knowledge is, so much the more excellent it is. Of all the men in the world I hate a drone most, that sucks the sweetness of other men's labors, but does no good himself; and will as soon teach Physic or Astrology to an Oak, as to a creature the center of whose actions is terminated in himself. Surely, surely, if God had not made the nature of man communicative, he would not have made one man to stand in continual need of another: but we see the contrary, and the sons of wisdom know how to pick out the meaning of God from it.

I have given you here all my Prognostications from the Decumbiture of the sick party: And although I ingenuously confess the greatest part of them will hold true, in a Horarie Question erected upon the sight of the Urine; yet this is my judgment at present, that next to the Nativity, the Decumbiture is the safest & surest ground for you to build your judgment upon; and you shall always find it by experience.

Together with this I have given you the presages of Hippocrates, all which never decline from the Zodiac of the sick person: And thus much I can say of them by experience, I never found one of them false. Make use of them both together; God has given you two eyes; why may you not look upon the Macrocosm with the one, and upon the Microcosm with the other? In both I desired to be as plain as I could, because all Artists are not Scholars.

Thus have you what I have done, and you know for whose sakes I did it. What now remains, but that you labor with might and main for your own goods, and the increase of your own knowledge to make experience of them? For as the diligent hand makes rich, so the diligent mind increases knowledge; and for my own particular, never fear, but during the time I am amongst the living, I shall never cease to do you good in what I may or can.

Spittle-fields, next door to the Red-Lion.

Nich. Culpeper.

note to readers 2

To The Reader

Excellent and true was that Motto of Hermes Trismegistus. *Quod est superius, est sicut inferius,* and this will appear to the eye of every one that deserves the name of a reasonable man, if he do but consider that his body is made of the same materials that the whole Universe is made of, though not in the same form; namely of a composition of contrary Elements. There is scarce a man breathing that knows his right hand from his left, but knows that if you set bottles of hot water to a man's feet, it will make his head to sweat; and the reason is the mutual harmony of one part of the body with another; why then as well should not the actions of one part of the Creation produce as well effects in another, that being also one entire body, composed of the same Elements, and in as great Harmonie? What's the reason that a man will do more for his brother then he will for a stranger? Is it not because he is formed by the blood of the same Mother, and begotten by the seed of the same Father? Why then should not the Celestial bodies act upon the Terrestrial, they being made of the same matter, and by the finger of the same God? He that will not believe Reason, let him believe Experience; he that will believe neither, is little better than an Infidel. I confess this way of Judicature has been desired by many; promised by some; but hitherto performed by none; which was the motive cause I now took the task in hand myself: In performing which, in many places I corrected the failings of my Author. What was frivolous I left out, as being unwilling to blot paper, and trouble your brains with impertinences: where he was too large, I abbreviated him: and where he was deficient, I supplied him both with Precept and Example. If there be any failings, consider,

1. Nemo sine crimine vivit.

2. That man nev'r breathed yet, nor never shall,

3. That did all well, and had no fault at all.

4. My failings (if any be) were not intentional, but accidental, together with this Astrological judgment, I have also given you the Judgment of Hippocrates. The rules whereof are drawn from the person of the sick, which although they have been often printed before, yet I have compared them with the original Copy, and brought them into a plainer method, so that you may have your desire at one single ingress. If you make use of both these ways together in judging of the disease, without a miracle you can hardly fail. If any find fault with the shortness of my rules, let them learn to walk worthy of those they have first; their own Experience will bring them more; he's but an apish Physician that builds all his practice upon other men's foundations: Man was born to look after knowledge, and in this particular you are set in the way how to find it, by one that desires to remain a friend to all honest and ingenuous Arts.

Nich. Culpeper.

note to readers 3

I promised a table of explanation of some hard words in one place of the book, but having looked over the book, I can find none but those at that place which can exceed almost the meanest capacity.

The words there are these three: Uvula, Gargarion, Columella, the signification of them is all one: I shall tell you,

1. What its substance and place is.

2. What its uses are.

The Uvula, Gargarion or Columella, choose you whether, is a red spongy piece of flesh sticking to the roof of the mouth near the throat. Its uses are,

1. To give pleasantness to the voice, therefore in hoarseness this is afflicted.

2. To stay the air that it pass not too fast upon the lungs; therefore, such as have gotten colds cannot sing well.

3. It hinders drink, and such liquid things as we eat, from coming out at our noses.

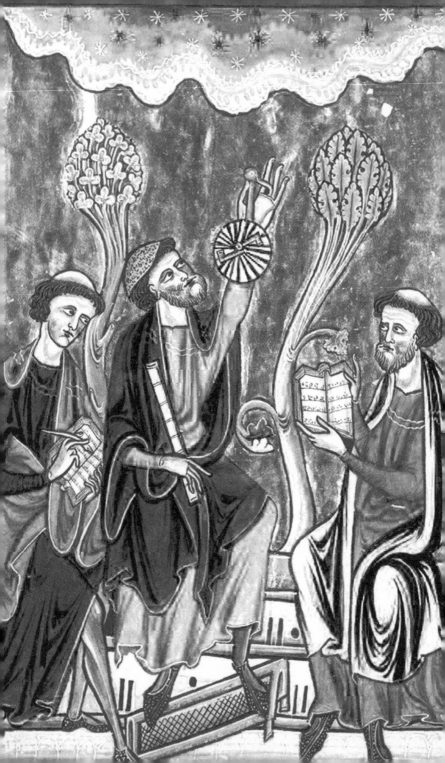

Introduction: Abraham Avenezra's[2], Of Critical Days

It is a palpable and apparent truth that God carries men to the principles of grace by the Book of the Creatures; for this beginning of Abraham Avenezra an Arabian Physician, and a singular Astrologer (whom the Priests of our times call a Heathen) savored of the things beyond Heathenism; for in this Treatise, *Of Critical Days*, he begins thus:

I entreat the Lord God, that he would enlighten my heart with his light and truth, so long as my Spirit remains in me, for his light is very delightful and good for the eye of my soul to see by; for so shall the night be enlightened to me as the day, neither shall the clouds shadow it; it shall not be like the light of the Sun by day, because it shall not be clouded, nor like the light of the Moon, because it shall never be diminished as her light is. God has made these lights as he has made man and he appointed the greater light to rule the day, and the lesser to rule the night; hence it appears, the Sun was made to rule the day, and not to give light to it only, as the Priests affirm: and the Moon was made to rule the night, not to give light to it only, as appears Gen. 1. because she has no light to give; also he has made the whole host of heaven, the fixed Stars and Planets, and gave them virtues, together with the Luminaries; but their virtues are not so great as the virtues of Luminaries; are neither is the virtue of the Moon so great as the virtue of the Sun, because she borrows her light from the Sun; also the whole host of heaven, that is, the fixed Stars move all in the same Sphere, and therefore their

2 Abraham Ibn Ezra, born around 1093 in Spain, was a Jewish scholar-philosopher-poet-astrologer.

distance is always the same the one from the other, and their latitude is always the same; but it is not so with the Planets; for their course is various, and so is their distance the one from the other, and so is their latitude; for sometimes they are upon the Ecliptic, sometimes North from it, sometimes South, sometimes Retrograde, sometimes direct, sometimes in conjunction one with another, sometimes in opposition, sometimes in other aspects; the reason of this is, because the Sphere of one is lower than the Sphere of the other, and the lower the Sphere is, the sooner they make their revolution.

The nearest to the earth of all the Planets is the Moon, and therefore her course is swiftest: and besides her difference in longitude and latitude, there happen other accidents to her which are not visible to other Planets; for sometimes she increases, sometimes decreases, and sometimes she is invisible or fails in light: the reason why the Planets are not seen horned as the Moon is because their distance is greater from us; all the Planets seem biggest when they are at their greatest distance from the Sun, or when they are nearest to the earth, according to Copernicus; also sometimes the Moon is Eclipsed, but not in the same manner as the Sun, for the Sun never loses its light, but is only shadowed from a particular people or place, by the body of the Moon; but the Moon Eclipsed totally loses her light; and the reason is, the Sun's light is his own, but the Moon is a borrowed light.

This being premised, consider that all things under the Moon universally, whether men, beasts, or plants, are changed, and never remain in the same state, neither are their thoughts and deeds the same: take counsel of your head, and it will certify you what I speak is true; and they are varied according to the various course and disposition of the Planets; look upon your own genesis, and you shall find your thoughts moved to choler, so often as the Moon transits the place where the body or aspect of Mars was in your genesis; and to melancholy when she does the like to Saturn; the reason is, because the Moon is assimilated to the body of man: whose virtue as well as her light increases and diminishes; for she brings down the virtue of the other Planets to the creatures, and to man if he lives upon the earth.

The Sun causes heat and cold, day and night, Winter and Summer; when he arrives to the house of his honor or exaltation, to wit, Aries, then the trees spring, living creatures are comforted, the birds sing, the whole creation rejoices, and sickness in the body show themselves in their colors; also when he arrives at his fall, to wit, Libra, the leaves of the trees fall, all creatures are lumpish, and mourn like the trees in October.

Also another notable experiment is, usually sick people are something eased from midnight to noon, because then the Sun is in the ascending part of the heavens; but they are most troubled when he is descending, that is, from noon to midnight.

The course of the Moon is to be observed in many operations both in the Sea and Rivers, Vegetables, Shellfishes, as also in the bones and marrow of men, and all creatures; also seed sown at the wane of the Moon grows either not at all, or to no purpose.

Also wise men have experiences of many virtues of the stars, and have left them to posterity: and Physicians in old times when they were minded to be honest, have found out the changes and terminations of diseases, by the course of the Moon; Wherefore the 7, 14, 20, or 21, 27, 28, or 29. Days of sickness are called Critical days, which cannot be known but by the course of the Moon; for let not your brain rest in the number of the days, because the Moon is sometimes swifter, sometimes slower.

As for such diseases as do not terminate in a month (I mean a Lunar Month) viz. the time the Moon traces round the zodiac, which is 27 days, some odd hours, some few minutes; you must judge of these by the course of the Sun; the day is not called Critical, because it is the seventh day from the decumbiture, as if the virtue lay in the number 7.

But because the Moon comes to the quartile of the place she was in at the decumbiture, it's no matter whether it be a day sooner or later.

When she comes to the opposition of the place she was in at the day of the decumbiture, she makes a second Crisis, the third when she comes to the second quartile, and the fourth when she comes to the place she was in at the decumbiture, and it's well she can make so many; being the reason of the difference of the Moon's motion in the difference of her distance from the Earth; for when the center of her circle is nearest to the center of the Earth, she is swift in motion; and hence it comes to pass that sometimes she moves more than 15 degrees in 24 hours, sometimes less than 12. Therefore, if she be swift in motion, she comes to her own quartile in six days; if slow, not in seven; therefore must you judge according to the motion of the Moon, and not according to the number of the days.

Know then that the Crisis', viz. upon a Critical day, the Moon being well aspected by good Planets, it goes well with the sick; if to ill Planets, it goes ill; but I know you would be resolved in one particular, which is, if the Crisis depend upon the motion of the Moon, and her aspect to the Planets; what is the reason, if two men taken sick at one and the same time, that yet the Crisis of the one falls out well, and not so in the other.

I answer, the virtue working is changed according to the diversity of the virtue receiving; for you all know the Sun makes the clay hard, and the wax soft; it makes the cloth white, and the face black; so then if one be a child whose nature is hot and moist, the other a young man, and the third an old man, the Crisis works diversely in them all, because their ages are different.

Secondly, the time of the year carries a great stroke in this business; if it be in the Springtime, diseases are most obnoxious to a child, because his nature is hot and moist; a disease works most violently with a choleric man in Summer;

with a melancholy man in Autumn; with a phlegmatic by reason of age or complexion in Winter.

Thirdly, to this I add, suppose at the beginning of a disease, the Moon was in the place of Mars, in the genesis whose nature is hot and dry, if the disease be of heat it mightily aggravates it; not so if it be of cold; and you shall seldom find two men that had Mars at one and the same place in the genesis at one and the same time, fall sick and the disease differ either at the middle or at the end.

Questions:

1. Put the case, the age of the people, and the season of the year be the same, and the disease be the same, would the Crisis be the same, yea or no?

2. I answer thus, their complexions may be different, the one hot and dry, the other cold and moist: If the diseases be hot and dry, the effect will not be so violent upon a cold and moist body, as it will be upon a hot and dry; the fire will sooner seize upon that which is hot and dry than that which is cold and moist.

3. Imagine the complexions to be the same upon both parties?

4. I Answer, that is impossible, there must be some difference upon complexions; for though they may be the same in the universal, yet in particulars there must needs be some difference, by reason of their different diet, exercise and climate, unless they be born and brought up together under one latitude.

5. Let us imagine they be all alike, yet diverse things may intervene and alter the Crisis; their nativities may not agree; for example, if the Moon be in the place of Saturn or Mars in the nativity, the disease is dangerous; not so if she be in the place where Jupiter or Venus was in then; or its possible Jupiter or Venus may hurt in the Nativities of such to

whose ascendents they are inimical or posited in the six or eight houses.

6. Again, Saturn may be Lord of the one nativity, and not of the other; and then he may hurt the one and not the other, whose nativity he is Lord of, for the Devil will not hurt his own; the like of Mars.

7. Innumerable such things may be added, as that the one may provide for the sickness beforehand, not the other, but it is needless.

Objection:

But then you will say, there can be no certainty at all found in the Crisis.

I answer, Astrologers pass judgment in two manner of ways in diseases.

The First we call universal, and so Saturn rules Consumptions, Mars fevers, Venus over women, Mercury over Scholars.

The Second is particular, and so the Seventh house has dominion over women, the ninth over Scholars.

Now no particular can destroy a universal; for example, if Venus be ill seated in a nativity, and the Lord of the Seventh well seated, we say the native shall generally incur evil by women, though some particular good may incur from them in like manner; judge in this case by the general signifiers of sickness, viz. Saturn and Mars.

But Secondly, if you can possibly get the Nativities you shall not err: And now give me leave to quote one experiment of my own. If the Nativities be one and the same, the Crisis will be one and the same: For example, I know three Children born at one and the same time (as the event proved) at five years of age they all three had Convulsions, whereby they were each of all three lame of one leg, the boys on the right leg, and the girls on the left; at fourteen years of age they died altogether in one and the same day of the small pox.

Thirdly, if the Nativity cannot be gotten, view the urine, and erect a celestial Scheme upon the sight of it, and if you have a decumbiture compass, the decumbitures with the celestial Scheme at the view of the urine, and you may judge clearly of the Crisis.

To proceed to the matter, if the Moon be strong when she comes to the Quartile or opposition of the place she was in at the decumbiture, viz. in her house or exaltation, the sick recovers if she be aspected to no Planet.

Judge the like of the Sun in Chronic diseases: but judge the contrary, if either of them be in detriments or falls; for there is as much difference between them as there is between the Zenith & the Narder; if the Moon be void of course at the beginning of a disease the sign is neither good nor bad. Look then to the sign ascending at the beginning of a disease, and let the Moon alone for a time.

If the Moon be angular at the decumbiture and in the Ascendent judge of her alone, and make use of no other signification; if she be [...] the Lord of the Ascendent with [...]

'Tis very dangerous when the Moon is Eclipsed, when she comes to the quartile or opposition of the place she was in at the decumbiture; so usually at such a time death turns Physician.

If in the beginning of a sickness the Moon is in a moveable sign, the sickness soon moves to an end one way or other; fixed signs prolong sickness, and common signs set a stop to the wisest brain in the world.

Also this is a certain rule, as sure as the Sun is up at noon day, that diseases of plenitude are very dangerous, when a man is taken sick upon a full Moon. Diseases of fasting or emptiness are most dangerous when a man is taken sick upon a new Moon. Let me entreat you to give Physic for a disease of emptiness when she is near the full. And for diseases of fullness when the Moon has lost her light.

Diminish a Humor when the Moon diminishes in light: Increase when she increases in light; Phlegm opposes Choler, Melancholy opposes Blood: 'tis none of the worst ways to diminish choler by increasing phlegm; a word is enough to the wise.

'Tis very bad when in the beginning of a sickness the moon is in a sign of the nature, if the quartile offending, naturally when she is in a fiery sign, amend a disease of phlegm; but if choler abounds, 'tis very good if she be in a watery sign; you may know by a penny how a shilling is coined.

If the moon be in conjunction or aspect with any Planet, and neither of them Latitude, the Crisis will be firm: if they differ much in Latitude the Crisis will be weak.

The Moon in conjunction with Saturn at the decumbiture shows long sickness; and if Saturn is slow in motion, so much the worse (and bad is the best) at all times in such a case.

If Saturn be retrograde when he comes to the opposition of the Sun beware of a Relapse.

If Saturn have North Latitude, be sure the sick is bound much in body. If the Moon be joined to a retrograde Planet, the sick vomits up his Physic.

Venus helps more in the sickness of young men and women than she does in old.

If the disease comes from heat, Venus helps more than Jupiter; if the disease comes more from cold, Jupiter helps more than Venus. If the disease comes of Love, there is not a more pestilent Planet in the heavens then Venus; then call help of Jupiter: in persecutions of Religion, Jupiter is little better than the Devil; call help of Venus in such a case.

Mercury accidental and strong, signifies good in diseases.

If Mars causes the disease, Venus helps more than Jupiter; if Saturn, then Jupiter more than Venus.

If in the beginning of a sickness the Moon is in conjunction with any fixed stars of the first magnitude, whose Latitude from the Ecliptic is but small, you may safely judge of diseases by the nature of that Star she is joined to; suppose he be of the nature of a Planet good or bad, take him according to his nature.

When the Moon is joined to any planet by body or aspect in the beginning of any sickness, if she aspect that Planet when she comes to the quartile or opposition of the place, the Crisis will be firm and stable, and will move no faster than a house, and will not be altered be it good or bad.

But if when she comes to quartile or opposition she meets with another Planet, be sure the disease changes either to better or worse, according to the nature of that star she meets withall.

And this will appear in the sick party, or else in the Physician, or in the course of Physick.

See what house the Planets she meets withall at the Crisis is lord of the decumbiture, and judge accordingly; and so a sick person may happen to have more wit than an old doting Physician.

If it be a fixed star of another nature to that fixed star she was withall at the decumbiture, it will not alter so much, or at least there will not be a universal alteration of the disease; and my reason is, because the fixed stars are so far from the earth. And the last the thing is, whatsoever is said of the Moon in acute diseases, will hold as true of the Sun in Chronic Diseases.

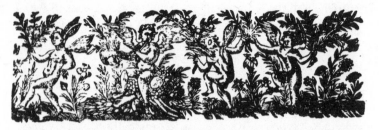

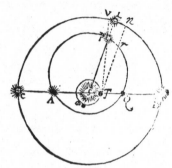

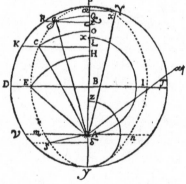

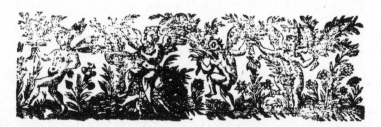

Astrological judgment upon Diseases; Or, A Methodical way to find out the Cause, Nature, Symptoms, and change of a Disease, together with the parts of the afflicted, the exact time of recovery, or dissolutions by the Decumbiture; Amplified by Examples.

The Basis of the Story was borrowed from Noel Duryet,[3] Cosmographer to the King of France and the most excellent Cardinal, the Duke of Richelieu.

'Tis confessed, in some places I have abbreviated him, in others corrected him; let another do the like by me: What I have done, I have done, and am not ashamed the world should see it. Through the never failing mercies of God, I had an opportunity put into my hands to finish this so much desired, so long wished for work; if there be any weakness in it, it is my own; if there be any excellency in it, give God the glory.

---

3 Noël Duret or Natalis Durret, born in 1590, was a French astronomer and mathematician.

He that writes ignominy upon the backside of another man's book, never setting forth any of his own, let the name of ignominy be branded, and not engraven upon his Sepulcher.

I would fain see the piss Prophets of this age deliver such a judgment of diseases by the Urine; he that can do so, *Erit mihi magnus Apollo*. Why do I trouble my head with the Physicians whose Covetousness or Laziness, or both, or something worse, will not suffer them to study those Arts which are essential to their Monopolized calling; but I will be silent; for their fall is approaching by reason of their pride, if he wrote true that writes, that pride goes before a fall, and a haughty mind before destruction: my Genius is too dull to commend my Author, or to give him the thousandth part of his due praise. I desire to be censured by Dr. Experience, who will give judgment without partiality and I hope 'tis no disparagement to Monsieur Duryat that I deliver him in my own Language.

The Definition of the word Crisis, as Use, Cause, Kinds, Division, and Difference.

Crisis, according to Galen, is a swift and sudden change of any disease, whereby the sick is either brought to recovery, or death; and a sick man can be brought to nothing else, unless you will make him a beast of a man.

For every swift and sudden change wherever it happens, whether in the Moon or the air, or sick body, Galen plays the man and calls a Crisis; and from this Crisis is Judgment given, whether the sick be like to live or die.

The word Crisis is a Greek word derived [...], which signifies to judge or discern, or pass sentence upon a thing: therefore Critical days are nothing else but days wherein a man may discern a disease, or give judgment upon it, be it good or bad, it matters not much; 'tis taken by a Metaphor from the Judicial Court to the Art of Physic, because 'tis something like to plead; man's cause for his life, and to labor acutely under a disease to be drawn by Inimical accusers before the judgment Seat, and to run the hazard of life, with a cruel and hostile Disease. Moreover there are three things requisite to a judicial Court: the Accuser, the Person indicted, and the Judge. So, likewise, are there three things by which the Art of Physic consists, and by which every cure is perfected: 1. The Disease, 2. Nature, and the Physician, which is nature's servant, or at least should be so; and 3. the accidents which manifest what the disease is, and stand as witness.

The cause of the Crisis is twofold; inward, outward; the internal cause is taken from its one proper principle, if you will believe Hippocrates; and that is double or two-fold; for either nature labors to expel the humor that causes the disease, or else the humor itself, being drawn to a place, and not fit for Excretion by its own weight or quality, burdens nature and sores break out. Hippocrates was but a man, and I am no more; a man, says he, is troubled when he is in a Fever, and the sign is horror, trembling, running hither and thither throughout the Microcosm; this is one internal cause.

The second internal cause. Others there be, 'tis no matter who, that ascribe the efficient cause of the Crisis to nature itself: Nature if she be strong, as 'tis pity but she should not, is a good Physician for all diseases; and concocts the humor which causes the disease, and separates that which is good from that which is bad; and having done so, prepares that which breeds annoyances for Excretion, and at last makes a shift to cast it out.

The external cause of the Crisis, is caused by an alteration of the air, whence ariseth an alteration of the breath a man draws in, from cold to heat, from dry to moist, or the contraries to them both.

For Hippocrates himself in his six Aphorisms, three Comments, and in his Treatise De [...], speaks in down dunstable language, that heat and moisture in the body, moves forward the Crisis: for diseases, some say he, come by ill diet, others by the air we draw in.

So then the diet as it breeds such and such humors in the body, is internal; but the air we draw in, is the external cause of the Crisis.

And now give me leave to leave my Author, and yet I will not forget him quite either. The Lord eternal in the beginning when he made the Creation, made it of a composition of contraries; discord makes a harmony as in Music; if the World be composed of a composition of contraries, various must needs be the disposition of man's life: Hence comes sometimes health, sometimes sickness, sometimes melancholy, sometimes choler to the body of man, and happy is that man that knows himself.

These qualities in man being altered by the various influences of the Stars, the Sphere of the one carrying a swifter motion than the Sphere of the other, then various must needs be the disposition of man's body.

The Luminaries carry the greatest strength in the heavens, and so do the time-servers in the State; and this needs not be doubtful to anybody, if you consider that the sound of a Drum or Trumpet incites a man to valor; and the sound of a Fiddle to dancing. Besides, other manifest effects of the Luminaries appear to our eyes. Who makes hours and days, and seasons in the year? Is it not the Sun? Who makes alterations in the air, in Plants, and in living Creatures? What is the reason that Oysters are fuller at the full moon than at the new? To the number of Oysters, join Crabs and Lobsters; nay the marrow in the body of Man; is it not the Moon? A man if he pleases, may say his right hand is his left, and a prating Priest may preach his pleasure, let Doctor Experience be judge. Now then we have brought the matter to this purpose, that the universal cause of the Crisis is the influence of the heavens: for the Celestial bodies either by heat, light, motion, or aspect, configuration, or all of them, or some of them, act not only in the four Elements, but Elementary bodies; for if they act in the one, they must needs in the other; and then by consequence in man, which is but compounded of Elements.

The earth is a great lump of dirt rolled up together, and by an only wise God hangs in the air; the Stars are no more, neither is the Moon; only what mettle the Sun is made of I know not.

If the bodies of men are Elementary, composed of Fire, air, Earth and Water; he must participate in one measure or other of all these Elements. The Elements being contraries, cannot always agree; hence comes the cause of health, sometimes of sickness, sometimes death itself; and Aristotle was half of my opinion when he wrote these words: "From the Rain and Dew of Heaven both good and bad things are caused to bud."

Kinds of Crisis

The kinds of Crisis are two; one in acute diseases, and they are to be judged by the Moon; the other in long and lasting, or chronic diseases, which are to be judged of by the Sun: For those Crises which come from their own proper principle, are from the internal cause depending only upon the motions of the Moon and her Configurations and aspects to the place she was in at the Decumbiture.

But you must note in acute diseases, the aspects or radiations of the Moon, to wit her Quartile or Opposition, are not taken from the Conjunction of the Moon to the Sun, as they are in Almanacs or Ephemerides, which is but the Father of an Almanac, but from the place in which the Moon was found at the Decumbiture, as shall appear by a few examples hereafter.

There are acute and Chronic diseases.

Of Acute diseases, some are simply acute, others are peracute, others are very acute, per-per-acute, or exceeding acute.

Tabula afcedetis et duodecim domorum

dies menfium	hore minuta	1 (7) g'cace g	2 (8) leo g	3 (9) leo g	4 (10) fgaittarg g	5 (11) fcoz g	6 (12) fagi g	dies menfium	hore minuta	1 (7) leo g	2 (8) leo g	3 (6) fgaittarg g	4 (10) libz g	5 (11) fcoz g	6 (12) capc g
1	0 0	12	3	26	20	0	7	1	1 53	5	29	25	21	28	1
2	0 4	13	4	27	21	1	8	2	1 56	5	30	26	22	29	2
3	0 8	13	5	28	22	2	9	3	2 0	6	1	27	23	30	3
4	0 11	14	6	29	23	3	10	4	2 4	7	2	28	24	30	4
5	0 15	15	7	30	24	4	11	5	2 7	8	3	29	25	1	5
6	0 19	16	8	1	25	5	12	6	2 11	9	3	30	26	2	5
7	0 22	17	8	2	26	6	12	7	2 15	9	4	1	27	3	6
8	0 26	17	9	3	27	7	13	8	2 18	10	5	2	28	4	6
9	0 30	18	10	4	28	8	14	9	2 22	11	6	3	29	4	7
10	0 33	19	11	4	29	9	14	10	2 25	12	7	4	30	5	8
11	0 37	19	12	5	30	9	15	11	2 29	12	8	5	1	6	9
12	0 41	20	12	6	1	10	16	12	2 33	13	9	5	2	7	9
13	0 44	21	13	7	2	11	17	13	2 37	14	9	6	3	8	10
14	0 48	22	14	8	3	12	18	14	2 41	14	10	7	4	9	11
15	0 52	22	15	9	4	13	18	15	2 44	15	10	7	4	9	11
16	0 55	23	16	10	5	14	19	16	2 48	15	11	8	5	10	12
17	0 59	24	17	11	6	15	20	17	2 52	16	12	9	6	10	12
18	1 2	25	18	12	7	16	21	18	2 56	17	13	10	7	11	13
19	1 6	25	18	13	8	17	21	19	3 0	17	14	11	8	12	14
20	1 01	26	19	13	9	17	22	20	3 3	18	15	12	9	13	15
21	1 13	27	20	14	10	18	23	21	3 7	19	16	13	10	14	15
22	1 17	28	21	15	11	19	24	22	3 11	20	16	14	11	15	16
23	1 20	28	22	16	12	20	24	23	3 15	20	17	15	12	15	17
24	1 24	29	22	17	13	21	25	24	3 19	21	18	16	13	16	18
25	1 28	30	23	18	14	22	26	25	3 23	22	19	17	14	17	18
26	1 31	30	24	19	15	23	27	26	3 26	23	20	18	15	18	19
27	1 35	Ω 1	25	20	16	23	27	27	3 30	23	21	19	16	18	20
28	1 38	2	25	21	17	24	28	28	3 34	24	22	20	17	19	21
29	1 42	3	26	22	18	25	29	29	3 38	25	23	21	18	20	22
30	1 46	3	27	23	19	26	29	30	3 41	26	24	22	19	21	23
31	1 49	4	28	24	20	27	30	0	0 0	0	0	0	0	0	0

Those which are simply acute, are finished in 8, 10, 11, 14, 20, or 21 days, and they are called Monthly diseases by some, and Lunary by others, and they are none of the greatest fools either; they are terminated in the time the Moon traces the 12 celestial signs of the zodiac, which is in 27 days, some odd hours, and some odd minutes.

Those acute diseases which suffer changes or degenerate, are to be judged of by an imperfect way; as for them sometimes they increase, sometimes they are remitted; they are as fickle as a weather Cock, according as the Moon meets with the beams either of good or evil Planets: and that is not all the trick they have neither. For sometimes they change out of acute diseases into Chronic diseases; and so a continued Fever may change into a Hectic Fever; or an intermitting Fever into a continued Fever; and these diseases terminate in forty days, very acute diseases, such as are concluded in 5, 6, 7, 8 days, among which are the Fevers the Greeks call [...], an inflammation of the Lungs.

In exceedingly acute diseases, they are such which end in three or four days at furthest, as Pestilencies, Apoplexies, etc.

Chronic diseases follow the motion of the Sun, and 'tis about nine days before the first Crisis appears; for in that time the Sun comes to the proper Quartile of the place he was in at the Decumbiture, as appears in Hectic Fevers, Dropsies: but when he comes to his Sextile, or Trine aspect of the place he was in at the Decumbiture, some motion appears whereby a man if he have any guts in his brains, may judge of the Crisis to come.

It falls out well, if the Sun be well aspected by good Planets, and worle if to evil Planets; and this holds true, if you consider it from the Nativity, throughout all the whole course of a man's life: for diseases are particularly attendants on a man's life, if Dr. Experience tell truth.

Moreover of the Crises, some are perfect, some are imperfect.

A perfect Crisis is, when the disease appears entirely and perfectly to be judged of; and this is sometimes hopeful, sometimes desperate; hopeful when there is great probability of health and recovery; desperate when there are palpable signs of death.

An imperfect Crisis is when the disease is changed upon every light occasion; and if Mars be Author of the disease, and in a sign of a double body, upon my life you shall not fail; for the Critis happens as true as the Weather-cock.

Your safest way then to judge of the disease is by the Aspects of the Moon to the Planets; when the Moon meets with the Inimical, or hostile beams of Saturn, or Mars, have a care of your Patient: And if you know what hinders, by the same reason, you may know what helps. Physicians in former, when they were wise, and minded the common good, and not their own gain, they distinguished the Crisis of diseases thus: Some were safe, some doubtful; some fit to be judged, and some not fit to be judged.

That Crisis is safe, which comes without great and pernicious aspects.

It is doubtful, suspicious, I had almost said dangerous, which comes with great pernicious aspects.

The disease is fit to be judged when signs of Concoction come the fourth day; and then certainly the Crisis will appear the 9th. The Moon moves not upon an equal motion; therefore you had best trust to her motion, rather than the days.

The Sun has domination in Chronic diseases, the Moon in acute; if you be a wise man, your judgment shall be as sure as the Sun, and that never fails without a miracle.

In times of yore, when knowledge was scant, men went a begging for it; and they that had gotten knowledge, monopolized it. A few glimpses of Adam's happiness in Paradise, which happiness all the World have been reaching after ever since.

They knew well enough the Moon moved so many degrees, in so many days: an evil Angel, I had almost said the Devil, perceiving there was want of knowledge in the World, goes and transforms himself into an Angel of light, and taught men to count the time by days: 'Tis no great marvel the Egyptians should worship Garlic and Onions for Gods, when we defy Christmas-day, though perhaps it may be cloudy.

What I have spoken, I have only spoken to show that it is the motion of Sun and Moon that produces the Crisis in diseases, and not the number of days.

I must return to the place I intended; Of days, some are called by their own name, Critical days; other are called Judicial days, and they are so called, because upon them, dame Nature and her Son Doctor Reason would make manifest what the disease is: and Doctor Experience tells me 'tis true.

Another time is called Intercidental, which is a time that falls out between the judicial days and Critical. Upon these Intercidental days, the disease is usually remitted; if so, then a good Crisis may be expected; if not, an evil. I shall explain these terms before I go further; a man falls sick, there is the first Crisis, let the cause of the disease be what you will; when the Moon comes to the same degree of the next figure she was in at the Decumbiture, there is the judicial days; for in that time the disease shows itself in its colors, with bag and baggage. When the Moon comes to her Sextile, it brings the Intercidental Day, and should mitigate the disease; if she do not, she is aspected to evil Planets: and if she be aspected to ill Planets, an ill Crisis is to be expected, and so the contrary; and you shall never find this fail.

The way to find out the Critical days, as also the Decumbiture, both by Ancient and Modern Writers.

Ancient Physicians, because they were ignorant of the motion of the Moon, though not of her operation, as many of our modern are, made their account by number of days; and in so doing, erred egregiously: And although Durate, my Author, counts their opinions, I hold it not worth time to recite men's failings: But of the certain term or time when the Critical days begin, I shall quote these few words. When any notable disease comes, if you would discern whether it tends to Health, Death, Mutation, or Continuance, it is necessary that you begin at the first punct of time of the invasion of the disease. This Galen says is very hard, if not impossible to find; 'tis taken *pro confesso*, that it may be easily known, when a man takes his bed in his sickness; but when the beginning of the sickness is, that's the question: For a lusty, stout man bears the disease longer, and is longer before he takes his bed, than a puny, weakly, sickly man is: a mere suspicion of a sickness, will send a faint-hearted man to bed; you may persuade him he is sick, whether he be or no.

Notwithstanding, this is most certain that in most acute diseases, as also in many other diseases, as the Falling sickness, Palsies, Apoplexies, Pluresies, etc. 'tis an easy thing to find out the beginning, or the precise time of the invasion of the disease.

The common opinion of such as are learned in Astrology is, and according to their opinion I affirm, that that moment of time is to be taken for the beginning of the disease, in which a man finds a manifest pain or hurt in his body: for instance, when a man has got a Fever, usually the head aches certain days before; this is not the Fever, but a Messenger or forerunner of the Fever; the true beginning of the Fever, is when the disease appears sensibly, or when a horror or trembling invades the sick, as does usually in the beginning of a Fever; that is the beginning of the disease, when the disease appears manifest to sense; And this was the judgment of Hippocrates, one of the honestest of Physicians: "And you shall find this always, that the more acute the disease is, the more manifest the beginning of it is to sense: yea so manifest, that it is almost impossible that the beginning should lie hid from any one that wants reason, if he have but sense."

Of the Sympathy and Antipathy of the signs and Planets.

Before we come to prognostic, we must know that there is a Sympathy between celestial and Terrestrial bodies, which will easily appear, if we consider that the whole creation is one entire and united body, composed by the power of an All-wise God, of a composition of discords.

Also there is friendship and hatred between one sign of the zodiac and another; for fiery signs are contrary to watery, and nocturnal to diurnal, etc.

The Planets are also friendly and inimical one to another; but in their friendship and enmity, whatever the matter is, I cannot agree neither with ancient nor modern writers: And when I cannot do so, I fly to Dr. Reason for advice; they hold Mars and Venus to be friends.

And what your opinion is of all the rest, you may find by Mr. Lilly's Introduction.[4] My own opinion, grounded upon reason, is this; that there are two causes of friendship and enmity, between Planets: essential and Accidental. Planets are essentially inimically three ways.

1. When their Houses or Exaltations are opposite one to the other; and so Saturn is an enemy to both Luminaries; Jupiter to Mercury, and contra Mars to Venus.

2. Planets are Inimical one to the other, when their temperatures or qualities are opposite; and so Jupiter is an enemy to Saturn, he being hot and moist, Saturn cold and dry: So Mars is enemy to Venus, he being hot and dry, she cold and moist.

3. Planets are Inimical when their conditions differ; so there is enmity to Sol and Jupiter, for he loves the Court, and he the Country. Jupiter is enemy to Mars, for he loves Peace and Justice, Mars violence and oppressions; Mars is enemy to Venus, for he rejoices in the field, she in the bed; he loves to be public, she plays least in sight. And thus you see in every respect, what a difficult thing it is to make Mars and Venus rationally friends.

---

4 William Lilly was an important English astrologer and contemporary of Culpeper.

Accidental inimicalness to Planets, is when they are in square or opposition, etc., the one to the other. Also Inimicalness must needs be in the signs; for if cold and heat, moisture and dryness, be inconsistent together in one and the same place, as your eyes will tell you, if you will but please to take a pail of water and throw it into the fire; then can they not be in one and the same place in the heavens. And if so, as is most true, then must some signs be cold, some dry, and some moist; one sign must needs cherish one quality more then another; and seeing the first qualities are adverse the one to the other, there is a necessity, that sometimes one must yield, and sometimes overcome: and this is the reason of the corruption, generation, and vicissitude of things.

Moreover the Moon constituted in a sign, commonly strikes upon the nature of the sign she is in: as if she be in a fiery sign, she stirs up Choler, etc.

Also as every Climate has two qualities, so has every celestial sign; the Aerial signs are hot and moist, the Earthly signs cold and dry, the Fiery signs hot and dry, the Watery signs cold and moist: And thus you see how the concords are made of discords; for Airy signs are joined to fiery by heat, and to watery by moisture: Watery are joined to airy by moisture, and to earthly by coldness: the Earthly are joined to the watery by coldness, and to fiery by dryness; this is an old true maxim of Philosophers; which I shall not at this time be captious against.

Besides, the congress and configuration of the Planets and fixed Stars is diligently to be heeded; of these, some are obnoxious and hateful; a Quartile and Opposition, as also the Conjunction of bad Planets; others are healthful, as Sextile and Trine, and Conjunction of good Planets; and indeed the chiefest part of Astrology consists in the due observation of configurations; for by these come alterations in things below, either to better or worse, according to the nature of the Planets or Stars that signify them: for when two Stars are joined with [...] aspected to one another, they seminate something in Sub-Lunary bodies according to their own nature; If dissention be between the stars, the sperm proves malicious and destructive, and tumultuous, even as the opposition of winds, especially the North and South winds, produce thunder, lightning and pestilential vapors, and this we find never fails, if the South-wind prevails, and the Moon and Mercury behold one another.

Thus you see a reason, if you know but what a reason is, or ever heard of such a thing, why diseases in the body of man are either exasperated, or remitted, according to the good or evil meeting of the Planets.

Of the Aspects, opposition is the worst of all, not by any contrariety, or diversity of nature of the Signs in which the oppositions fall out, but in respect to the Planets themselves opposing, which being at greatest distance are most inimical; they being in a posture to outface one another, and this is the most principal cause of enmity.

A Quartile is inimical, because the Stars so aspected be in signs of contrary nature; as Sol in Aries; Luna in Cancer, the aspect is hateful, because Aries is hot and dry, Cancer cold and moist; Aries masculine, Cancer feminine; Aries diurnal, Cancer nocturnal.

And now by the leave of my Author, and also of the great Ptolomy himself, and of all the sons of Art this day living, who build their judgment upon Doctor Tradition, and not upon the sound principles of Doctor Reason; if this be the original of the enmity of a square aspect, as is agreed upon on all sides:

Then, Why do they hold that a Quartile in Signs of long ascensions is equivalent to a Trine; and a Trine in Signs of short Ascensions as pernicious as a Square? Put the rest of the nonsense into the bundle: and when you have done, look upon it a little while, and when you have viewed it a little, tell me, I pray, does the longness or shortness of the ascensions add or take away anything from the quality of the signs?

Is not this the way, the only way, to bring the Art into a Labyrinth, if not into a confusion? In truth in my opinion it is; This I will confess, and give you my reason for it when I have done; one square is not so bad as another; as from Aries to Cancer is worse than from Cancer to Libra, because the Signs Cancer and Libra are in better harmony, as agreeing in passive qualities; namely, moisture, whereas Aries and Cancer disagree totally. By this rule you may find out the rest.

Also this I affirm and will prove it when I have done, that some Semisextiles are worse than some Quartiles; for Pisces is more inimical to Aries than Capricorn; first because it is the twelfth sign from him, and, besides, disagrees more in qualities.

A Sextile Aspect is good, because the Signs which are in Sextile the one to the other are both of the same active quality, both of a sex, both of a time, for example, Aries and Gemini are both masculine, both Diurnal; Taurus and Cancer are both cold, both Feminine, both Nocturnal; but because they differ all in passive qualities, it is not altogether so friendly as trine aspect is; for that consists altogether of signs of the same nature, sex, quality and time, and are correspondent the one to the other every way.

A Conjunction or Synod is the strongest of all, and cannot properly be called an aspect. A Conjunction of good Planets with good is exceeding good: It is good in the highest degree. A conjunction of bad Planets with bad Planets is as bad, as the former was good. A conjunction of good Planets with bad is no ways commendable. I have now done, if you will be pleased but to take notice, that the conjunction of all Planets with their Sun is bad, because the Sun who gives them their efficacy, takes it away at such times. I could be Critical at this, but I shall forbear it at this time.

The way of finding out the Critical and Judicial days by a Figure of eight houses.

This is the method of Hippocrates, and from him Galen used, and it is to be done in this manner.

1. Make your scheme of eight equal parts.

2. Search out the sign, Degree, and Minute the Moon was in at the beginning of the sickness.

3. Place the sign degree & minute the Moon was in at the beginning of the sickness upon the cusp of the first house, as though that were ascending at the time.

4. Add 45 degrees to this, you need not regard the latitude of the Region, for it is of no use in Critical Figures, but take the degrees barely from the Ecliptic, when you have added forty five degrees to the place of the Moon at the decumbiture, the point of the zodiac answerable to that shall make the cusp of the second house.

5. 45 degrees more added to that will bring you to the Cusp of the third House, to which when the Moon comes, she comes to the quartile of the place she was in at the decumbiture, and this makes the first Crisis.

6. 45 degrees more added to this, makes the 4th house; 45 degrees more added to that points out the place of the true opposition of the Moon to the place she was in at the decumbiture, and this makes the second Crisis. The second quartile of the Moon to her own place at the decumbiture, makes the third Crisis: And the fourth is when she comes to the same sign, degree and minute that she was in at the decumbiture.

The time or hours noted betwixt the Crisis are called the Judicial times; or such times wherein a man may judge what the disease is, or what it will be; remember this all along in such kinds of judgment; And do not forget not to number the time by days as the ancients did; for they were either ignorant, or regardless of the course of the Moon; for the Moon comes to the Judicial or Critical days, sometimes sooner, sometimes later, as she is either swifter or slower in motion.

Now the time called Critical is always evil, because of the contrariety of the sign the Moon is in then to the sign she was in before, or the contrariety of her nature to the opposite place: At such a time there arises a controversy or battle as it were, between the disease and nature; the Moon maintains nature in acute diseases: And now you have the reason why, that if she be afflicted upon a Critical day by the bodies or ill beams of Saturn or Mars, or the Lord of death, which is always Lord of the eighth House, and sometimes the Lord of the Fourth House, will serve the turn if he be malevolent, because the fignisies the grave, the disease increases, and sometimes the sick dies: But if the Moon at the time of the Crisis beholds the Lord of Ascendent or the fortunes fortunately, health ensues; for the malady is vanquished and routed in the conflict.

If the disease terminates not upon the first Crisis, see how the Moon is configured on the second Crisis, and judge then by the same Rules.

If it terminates not then either, as sometimes such a thing happens, view the third Crisis, and judge by that the same way; if your judgment balanced by reason, and the former rules, certify you the disease will not end one way nor other, neither in health nor death; see what you can say to the Moon when she returns to the place she was in at the decumbiture, which is about twenty-seven days, eight hours, and some few minutes; and see how the Moon is then seated, and to what Planets she is configured then: And this of necessity must be the end of all acute diseases.

Thus you see an acute disease can last but a month at longest; not one in a hundred lasts so long, not one in twenty lasts above half so long.

If the disease end not then, the acute disease is turned into a Chronic disease: And all Chronic diseases must be judged of by the Sun. The rules of judging of Chronic diseases by the Sun are the same by which we judge of acute diseases by the Moon.

As for Judicial days, which fall out just in the midst betwixt the Critical days, I shall pass them by at this time, because I fancy not this way of judgment by a Figure of eight houses; yet I shall not so pass them by, but that I shall remember them in the Treatise.

The former rules illustrated by an example.

A certain man fell sick of an acute disease at Paris in France, Anno 1641, Jan. 12, about eight of the clock in the afternoon, at which time the Moon was posited in Aquarius, 10. 19. This I place in the Ascendent.

To this Aquarius 10. 19. I add 45 degrees; the product is Pisces 25. 19., which makes the first judicial time;

To which adding 45 degrees more, it will bring you to Taurus 10. 19. to which place when the Moon arrives she comes to the exact quartile of the place she was in at the decumbiture, and makes the first Crisis.

Add 45 degrees to that, and it produces Gemini 25. 19., which is the second judicial time.

If you would know when the second Crisis comes about, it is but only Adding 45 degrees to that, and you will find the result to be Leo 10. 19. just the place opposite to the Moon at the decumbiture. The remainder are found out in the same manner.

When you have done so, it is no more but this:

First, seek the time when the Moon comes to Taurus 10. 19., and you shall find it comes upon the 19 of Jan. about eight of the Clock at night.

Secondly, View first the face of heaven, secondly the position and configuration of the Planets one with another at the same time.

A Synopsis, or joynt view of the Calculation.			
Critical dayes.	Moons motion.	Time of Incidence.	Lunar ſtate, according to the Decumbiture, her aſpects; as alſo the mutual aſpects of the Planets.
Decumbiture. Judicat. 1.	January 1. 2. ♒ 10. 19. ♓ 25. 19.	D.H.M. 12.8. 0. P. M. 16.5.43.A.M.	☽ ad ⚹ ♂ ad ♀ ♂ ♄ ☿ ☉ ♃ ☿ ☐ ☉ ♂ ☽ wagnâ, no Criſis to be expected.
1. Criſis. 2. Judicial. 2. Criſis.	♉ 10.19. ♊ 25. 10. ♌ 10.19.	19. 8.0. P.M. 23.2.36.P.M. 27.5.50.A.m.	☐ ♂ ♀, ☽ wagnâ. ☽ ad △ ♄ Threatens an ill Criſis. ☽ wagnâ, an ill Criſis,
3. Judicial. 3. Criſis.	25. 19. ♍ ♏ 10. 19.	30.3.44. P.M. February, 2.9. 1.P.M.	☽ ad △ ♄ ♃ A good Criſis to be hop ☽ ad △ ♀, he recovers.
4. Judicial. 5. Criſis.	25 19. ♐ 10.19. ♒		

A Synopsis, or joint view of the Calculation.

The History of this observation is of a certain person who by reason of great weariness in a journey, was surprised with a fever, at the time before mentioned; together with his fever he had a Cough and a Pleurisy; The fever came to a [...]. I never read of this name in Galen that I remember; I take it both by Monsieur Duryet's description, and also by his Figure of Heaven, to be the very same which Galen calls [...].

The original of this disease is Choler putrified with the blood in the veins, and is the most violent of all fevers. The night after the decumbiture this fever appeared; although on the third day all snaking left him, yet felt not the Patient the least intermission, the Moon being in Aquarius 10. 19. Aquarius being also a sign of infirmity, the Moon's being in Sextile to Mars applying to Venus and Saturn, Mars afflicting the Sun with a Quartile, as also Jupiter and Mercury who were in combustion.

The 16th day of the same month of January, the disease increased, at which time the moon came to a Semi-Quadrat making the first judicial time. And meeting then with never an aspect, the Crisis could be expected no other than doubtful and unfortunate.

The 19th day of the same Month at eight of the clock in the afternoon, the first Crisis came about some little sweat the diseased had. And if I may be bold to leave my Author for a little time, if you view the presages of Hippocrates, which you shall find at the latter end of this Book, the words run thus, or to this purpose: "It is very hopeful when a man sick of a fever sweats upon a Critical day." However, my Author confesses that both his Cough and his pain in his side left him, though his Fever still remain, nay increased; by reason of the Quartile of Mars and Venus at the same time Mercury being Lord of the Ascendent at the Decumbiture. Also, it is worth noting, that the Moon being in Aquarius at the decumbiture, and comes to Taurus at the first Crisis, both Taurus and Aquarius are signs of infirmity; yet you see the Pleurisy left him, the Moon being strong in her exaltation, though void of course.

I pass by my Author's infirmities in this and other things.

January 23. When the Moon by transit made the second judicial time, she was afflicted by the Trine of Saturn, which prognosticates cause enough of fear in the second Crisis.

January 27. At 5:50 in the morning, the Moon came to the true opposition, to the place she was in at the decumbiture, she being then without any Aspect, either good or evil; this brought no hopes to the sick man of cure at that time; and indeed the sick was at that time very bad; yea, so bad that his Physicians were in doubt whether he would live or die.

January 30. At 3 hours 44 minutes after noon, comes about the third judicial time, at which time the Moon was in Trine to Jupiter, which gives strong hopes that a healthful and propitious Crisis would ensue; and oh it did; for upon

February 2, at nine a clock after noon, the Moon coming to 10 degrees, 9 minutes of the Scorpion, where she made the second Quartile to the place she was in at the decumbiture, and the third Crisis she applied to the Trine of beautiful

Venus: his fever began to leave him, and he began to attain his pristine health.

By this one example you may see the wonderful harmony and consent of diseases with the motions of the heavens, which that it may appear more clear, and be visible to all, unless it be to such as are so blind they will not see, my Author adjoins a rational Figure of the decumbiture, and gives his judgment upon it.

An astrological judgment upon the face of Heaven at the Decumbiture.

The chief signifiers of this Figure are the Ascendent and Mercury Lord of it, Retrograde in Capricorn, a moveable sign in the 5th House of the Heaven, and in the House of Saturn.

The 6th house and his Lord Saturn in Aquarius, in the 6th house strong and potent.

The Moon in the 6th house upon the cusp of it; Sol in the 5th House with the Lord of the eighth, afflicted by the Quartile of Mars in a fiery sign; this plainly shows a disease of Choler.

Jupiter in a moveable sign in the 5th House, who rules the stomach, Liver and Sides, combust and in Quartile to Mars stirred up a Pleurisy, and Mercury afflicted showed a dry Cough. Hence it appears that Monsieur Duret was no Physician; for if he had, he would easily have known that a Pleurisy never comes without a dry Cough; the most excellent of men may have failings.

The Moon in Aquarius applying to Saturn at the beginning of the disease, shows the disease comes of weariness, according to the Doctrine both of Hippocrates and Hermes; but here arises another question; Shall the disease be long or short? This is answered thus, a fixed sign upon the cusp of the 6th House shows the length of the disease.

Saturn in the 6th House shows no less, but tells the same tale.

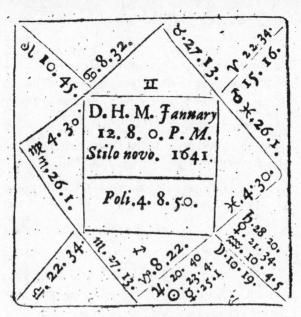

A Rational Figure upon the Decumbiture

Again Saturn Lord of the 6th, stronger than the Lord of the Ascendent, shows a violent increase of the disease.

Seeing Mars in a fiery sign afflicts both Luminaries, the Sun by a Quartile and the Moon by a Sextile; hence we may safely gather that Saturn and Mars are Authors of the disease, and to part stakes between them, the one made it violent, the other continuing.

Give me leave now a little to pass my judgment upon this Figure: When first I viewed the Figure, upon the first blush I admired the man should live; the Lord of the Ascendent being combust, and applied to the Sun, Mars casting Antiscion to the Sun, the Moon upon the Cusp of the 6th, *cum multis aliis*; the only reason that I could find of the life were these:

1. Saturn and Mars are both strong, and neither of them Lord of Death, though both of them of the sickness; then will they both of them show themselves like potent enemies, that are able to hurt their foe, but scorn it; though they are

enemies to life, yet they are honorable enemies, because strong.

2. The Moon implies not immediately to Saturn, but to the body of Mercury, who is Lord of the 10. which shows the disease might be cured by Physic if a wise Physician had it in hand.

3. There is a Reception between the Sun and Mars which ties the Sword of Mars from killing.

4. Venus beautifies the signification of the 6th house, almost as much as Saturn deforms it.

5. Neither Saturn nor Mars behold the Ascendent, and that's good.

6. The disease came by the man's own misguiding himself, because the Lord of the 12th and Ascendent are together.

7. The Moon applies to a fortune which has triplicity in the Ascendent, though in an ill House.

8. I am confident the man journeyed again so soon as he was well. First, because Mars, Lord of the end, is near the House of Journeys at the decumbiture; secondly, because the Moon applies to the Lady of the third House at the decumbiture, which is Venus.

The way to set a Figure of 16 Houses.

The way of setting this Figure differs nothing from the former, save only that the Heavens are divided into twice as many parts. The manner of erecting it, is this; the true place of the Moon being taken at the decumbiture, place that upon the Cusp of the Ascendent, as though it were ascending at the time, to which add 22 degrees 30 minutes, and you have the first intercidentall time 22. 30 being added to that show the first judicials time; as many more being added to that show the second intercidentall time; and as many added to them brings about the first Crisis; this shall be clearly showed in this Example. The Sun a Figure of Crisis in 16.

A Synopsis, or joynt view of the Calculation.			
Critical dayes.	Moons motion.	Time of Incidence.	Lunar state, according to the Decumbiture, her aspects, as also the mutual aspects of the Planets.
Decumbiture. Judicat. 1.	January 1, 2. ♒ 10. 19. ♓ 25. 19.	D.H.M. 12.8. 0. P. M. 16.5.43. A.M.	☽ ad ✶ ♂ ad ♀ ♂ ♄ ♂ ⊙ ♃ ☿ □ ⊙ ♂ ☽ vacuá, no Crisis to be expected.
1. Crisis. 2. Judicial. 2. Crisis.	♉ 10. 19. ♊ 25. 10. ♌ 10. 19.	19. 8. 0. P.M. 23.2.36. P.M. 27.5.50. A.m.	□ ♂ ♀. ☽ vacuá. ☽ ad △ ♄ Threatens an ill Crisis. ☽ vacuá, an ill Crisis.
3. Judicial. 3. Crisis.	25. 19. ♍ ♏ 10. 19.	30.3.44. P.M. February, 2.9. 1. P.M.	☽ ad △ ♄ ♃ A good Crisis to be hoped. ☽ ad △ ♀, he recovers.
4. Judicial. 4. Crisis.	25. 19. ♐ 10. 19. ♒		

A Synopsis of the Calculation

The History of this second observation is of a certain religious person, some Monk or Fryer a hundred to one else; who in 1640, December the ninth, stilo novo, was taken with a fever and shivering at eight of the Clock in the morning; the next day the shivering left him, the fever remaining; the fever seeming like a Hemitriters, or double tertian, or a Causus, which is a continual burning fever; which of them soever it was, this is certain, it arose from some choleric matter.

The second day it had another access, and the third worse than that.

The place of the Moon at the decumbiture was in a preterite trine of Saturn. The Moon applied to the Sextile of Mercury, Venus, and Jupiter.

The Fifteenth day of the same month of December appears the first Crisis; and though to sweat well many medicines were applied, and those powerful, yet the fever gave not way an inch, because the Moon applied to Mars, and the Sun to Saturn; though by good aspects; neither was it mitigated till the eighteenth day; at which time the Moon applied to Mercury, Venus, and Jupiter.

Here was that Aphorism of Hippocrates ratified, Chap. 5. Aphor. 15. that if the Moon be just afflicted at the decumbiture, yet if she be with the beams of the Malevolents at the Crisis, a good Crisis is not to be expected, but health will be staved off.

A Rational Figure upon the Decumbiture.

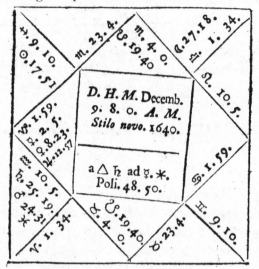

An Astrological judgment upon the Figure.

I confess in this judgment my Author is very faulty; he is dead, and I shall not make known his faults to my brethren the communality of England: however, this is true.

1. In this figure, Capricorn is upon the cusp of the ascendent; and it is a moveable sign; therefore, the disease is likely to be short.

2. Saturn, Lord of it, is very potent and strong in his own house, and swift in course, there's a Second Argument.

3. Both fortunes in the ascendent may well make up a third.

4. The moon applying to the fortunes, makes up a fourth; this is enough; only the Quartile of the Sun and Mars shows the sickness of Choler.

I could give you mine own observations upon this disease, if I would; but I let it alone and leave every man to his own heuretes.

How to set a Figure of twelve Houses for the Crisis.

This seems to me to be the most rational of all the rest, and it is the most easily and readily done; and it may be that's the reason my Author left it out, though he promised it. And indeed the ways of God are all easy, very easy. 'Tis the ways of men that are crabbed and difficult.

I shall first of all show you the way how to do it, secondly give you an example of mine own upon it.

First of all, if you would know how to make such a critical a figure upon a decumbiture, make you a Figure after the vulgar form; then note what sign, degree, and minute the Moon is in at the decumbiture, set that sign, degree, and minute on the ascendent, and thirty degrees to that, and the same degree and minute of the next sign will be upon the Cusp of the second house; the work is as easy walking upon and down without a staff, as I shall by and by make appear by an example.

Then be pleased to take notice, that the first house is the decumbiture; the second the judicial time; the third the intercidental; which word Dr. Phage of Midburst in Sussex, in his Book called *Speculum aegrotorum,* so sillily translates Mortals, mistaking the word Caedo to kill, for Cado to fall; wherein the man most egregiously showed his deficiency, both in Scholarship and Physic; yet this commendation I'll give him, his heart was more free to do good than his brain was able.

The fourth house brings the first Crisis about; and when you are come to that begin again as you did before; you may see the way without a pair of spectacles by the decumbiture, what I have quoted: you may take it *pro confesso*, if you please, that I have many decumbitures by me; but I want time to insert them, or if I did not, I would not blot paper with them.

Be pleased to accept this one in lieu of all the rest.

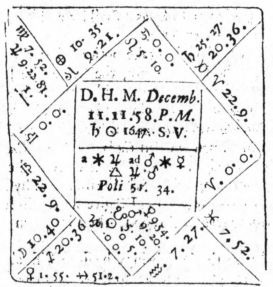

A Rational Figure on the Decumbiture.

This unhappy creature being untowardly matched with an unnatural husband; came up to London and lived in a service; and in her service was surprised with a furious disease at the time, and under the face of heaven before noted.

I shall first give a rational judgment of the Figure, and afterwards treat the Crisis.

The Person of this young woman is signified by Venus in Sagittarius; and truly I believe she was an upright dealing creature; that the cause of her disease lay hid, or at least very obscure; is plainly signified by so many Planets being under the earth.

That she procured her own disease, because the Lord of 6th is in the twelfth. As also because the Lord of the ascendent is disposed by a Planet in the 12th.

Pisces is the Cusp of the 6th. Her disease came by wet taken at the feet. Jupiter in Virgo gave corruption in blood, and infirmities in the bowels; with what they were, more anon.

Venus with the Scorpion's heart shows a violent fever; neither proved it to be any less.

The Sun and Mars in the Fourth house with the Dragon's-tail in Quartile to the ascendent, show violence in the disease, danger of poison and an ill end of it; her Physician is signified by Mars, which was a French quake which lay in the house, and he was like Mars in Capricorn, as a Pomewater is an Apple.

He was also troubled with sore eyes, a man of forlorn fortunes: view the position of Mars, and you shall easily see the reason without a pair of spectacles.

The position of Mars in the Fourth combust with the Dragon's-tail, and in the Quartile of the ascendents; First, clouded his judgment; secondly, corrupted his practice; thirdly set hard for her life.

'Tis a sad thing when the Lord of death must be the Physician in the disease.

Her disease was the smallpox in which being exceedingly bound in body, not going to stool in a week together and above; he applied her all that time with strong purges, (oh acute Physician) never one of them working nor so much as coming from her, though there was Scammony in every one of them, that had not I so soon as I knew of it persuaded her Nurse to give her a Glister every day, she had absolutely perished: her purges increasing her fever, and poisoning her body; and this I am confident was the reason, both of her being so much disfigured by her disease. And of her Aches and swelling in the knees (for Mars was in Capricorn) which continued upon her until her dying day, which followed about a year and a half after.

Neither was her Doctor's judgment one jot inferior to his practice; for in the beginning of the disease (viz. the next day after) she fell sick; I came accidentally to the house, and found all the household weeping; every one that could eat an egg shed a tear. A Joiner was busy pulling down the bedsteads, the whole household preparing for a flight, with bag and baggage.

And what was the reason think you? The Doctor had passed a wild piece of Nonsense, that she had got the pestilence, and was full of the tokens; up run I to see the Creature; I found her in a strong fever, that's true; but I could see no tokens, unless 'twere tokens of the Doctor's ignorance. I demanded the time of her falling sick, which she very exactly gave me: and having taken the pains to erect the figure, I did what I could to cherish up her spirits. I told her my judgment was that she would live; I certified the household that she had no such disease as the Pestilence; much less any tokens; and thus whoever lost, the Joiner he got money by the bargain on both hands, First, pulling the bedsteads and tables to pieces, and for setting them together again: and thus you see 'tis an ill wind that blows nobody no profit.

I have but two questions to answer, and then I come to the Crisis.

1. Will she live or die?

2. Will her sickness be long or short?

To the first of these I answer, that Mars is Lord of death, and also an afflicting Planet, in trine to the Lord of the Sixth. And in Sextile to the Moon, he with the Sun are in Quartile to the Ascendent; this is all the Signs of death, that is besides the great sign (viz.) her Doctor swore she would die, and could not possibly live, having, as the Cox-combe said, not so much of her lungs left, as amounted to the quantity of three of her fingers, a likely tale for sooth was it not?

I was a diligent observer of every passage in this sickness; and I found it always true, that during her sickness, the moon by transit to the body, or beams of Mars afflicted her sorely.

But not so to the beams of Saturn, for that only possessed her body with coldness and chillness.

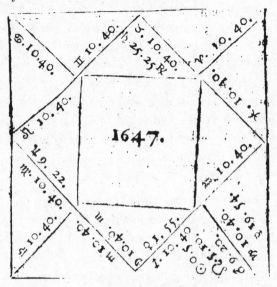

A Figure of Crisis.

That she should live is very clear; the Moon being with the Sextile of Jupiter, and the Lord of the Ascendent no way afflicted, save only by the Scorpion's heart.

To the Second Question, namely, whether her disease should be long or short?

The Angles being all Cardinal, and the Moon swift in motion, and in Sextile to Jupiter, show a short sickness; the Lord of the Ascendent, and the Lord of the Sixth, being both stationary, prolong the disease.

And indeed though the disease taken under the notion of acute, were long, yet taken according to reason, it is shorter than could be imagined.

The first judicial time is when the moon comes to Sagitarius, 10. 40. It's called a judicial time because at that time the disease appears in his colors that a man may know what it tends to.

The second time, which you may find upon the third House in the Critical Figure, is called intercidental, because it falls between judicial and Critical times: and upon this intercidental time, there is usually some remission of the disease, that so nature may have time to rally up her forces against her encounter, with the disease on her Crisis. And according as it falls out upon the intercidental day, either to good or bad, so a good or bad Crisis may be expected: But to return, the Moon comes to Sagittarius, 10. 40. upon the 14 of December, about half an hour after six in the Morning. If you please but to set the figure, you shall find she is just upon the Cusp in the ascendent, newly separated from the body of Venus, and the Quartile of Jupiter; now the smallpox came out, and not till now.

The first intercidental time happens when the Moon comes to 10. degrees 40 minutes of Capricorn, the place where Mars was at the Decumbiture, and now the applies to his body, having newly left the Trine of Jupiter. If you please to set the Figure, the time was December 16, 1 hour, 24 minutes, p.m. Saturn is upon the Cusp of the ascendent: about this time she got cold.

And I am of the opinion that the ascendent and sixth House being earthly signs at this time: and the Moon in Conjunction with Mars in another earthly sign, does clearly show her being bound in body. This day, which should have mitigated her disease, increases it; and now her Dr. (if I may call him so without a Solecism) begins to play the antique, I had almost said the mad man. Now he exercises her purging faculty, and leaves his wits abed and asleep with his last night's Mistress. Sure I am, a Physician would admire to hear Scammony given to a Creature that had the smallpox coming out upon her: To conclude, a very ill Crisis is threatened.

The first Crisis comes about upon the 18th of December, three quarters of an hour past 11 at night: the face of heaven is not much altered from what it was at the Decumbiture. The Moon separates from the Sextile of Venus Lady of the ascendent, and applies to the Quartile of Saturn; and had Dr. Dunce only judged she would have died now, as indeed he did, he might have been pardoned although he had fail'd; but alas, he, poor man, had little skill in times and seasons; his skill was employed to know a woman from a man, when he had got her in bed.

He did not only say, but also swore, that she would die about the intercidental time, though such a thing be seldom seen in a man's age: but let us to our Art, and let the Doctor's ignorance alone.

You shall find if you please to set the position of Heaven, the Scheme almost the same with that of the Decumbiture. The Moon carries the beams of the Lady of the ascendent to the Quartile of Saturn. The Sun and Mars cast hot full beams to the ascendent; and indeed my own opinion is that had the Moon applied to Mars, as she did to Saturn, it had killed her.

Howsoever, the premises considered, it is clear, that this is likely to be the time of greatest danger in all her sickness; and so indeed it was: Now must the disease needs be strongest, nature weakest: and if this time be passed, the bitterness of death is past indeed at this time. The Combate was sore, she distracted, senseless, the smallpox began to fall down; and with all, strength almost spent: but above all, the Doctor swore she could not live while morning.

Rational hopes of her life are the dignities of Saturn in the ascendent, but especially the Trine of the Sun and Jupiter upon that day. It is the opinion of the learned in this Art; that let the Significators of life or death be seated or disposed as badly as they can be; yet if the Sun be in Conjunction or good aspect with Jupiter, the sick will live; and truly so did she, almost to admiration.

But some will ask, and 'tis a question worth the answering; that if the Sun and Jupiter preserve life, as you say, when they are so seated: what's the reason men die at that time? For we see men die daily;

to this I answer briefly, that truly in the nativity of some people, Jupiter is the killing Planet; and in the sickness of sick persons, Jupiter will as soon kill, as Saturn and Mars; every Planet must do his Office: I proceed, the second judicial time comes about the 21st of December, at noon, or a very little after; at which time Mars is Lord of the ascendent strong, and in his exaltation.

The Moon having left the Sextile of the Sun, applies to his Sextile. The face of heaven is quite and clean altered from what it was at the Decumbiture, a manifest sign of some chance. Besides, though Saturn be in the ascendent, and Mars in the 10th House; yet Jupiter is in the 6th; therefore, some good may be hoped: I do not know that it is besides the rule of Art, if I should affirm that as Mars in the 4th House of the Decumbiture kept her Doctor's (you may call it) folly or madness (which you please) close; so now in the 10th house reveals it. Now, and not till now, did I know of her Doctor's frantic course of Physic, and of her not going to stool; from this time she took a Glister every day till she amended.

The second Crisis comes about upon the Sun, the 26 of December about one hour after noon; at which time the Moon is strong in her own exaltation, and applies to the Trine of the Sun and Mercury. At this time her fever left her, and she began to recover: And upon the third Crisis, which happened upon the first of January, she went abroad.

Certain precepts premised before the Prognostics.

First of all, take notice that the Signifiers of Diseases are to be taken under these two notions. 1. General, or more principal. 2. Particular, or less principal; The general or more principal are these: the Sun, the Moon, and the Ascendent; of these the Sun is most principally to be looked upon in Chronic diseases, the Moon in acute.

1. Signifiers of particular or less principal are these:
    • The Lord of the Ascendent.

- The sixth House.

- The Lord of the sixth House.

- The Planets in the ascendent or sixth House.

- Saturn and Mars; for they naturally hurt the body, whatsoever the matter is.

2. The sixth House and its Lord, and the Planets in it, if there be any there, best describe the nature of the disease usually, nay always, if they afflict either of the Luminaries, or the Lord of the ascendent.

3. The aspects of the Moon to the Planets are always to be noted; for they still produce something to the sick, but especially upon Critical and Judicial days; for you shall find this a certain truth, even as certain as the Sun (and he never fails without a miracle), that when the Moon passes by the bodies of Jupiter or Venus, or their aspects, especially their good ones, if they be not Lords of death, remits the most desperate Symptoms in a sickness, and gives the sick some ease; as also the bodies, or any aspect of Saturn or Mars exasperates a disease, and spoils the most hopeful Symptoms.

4. Here then you have one way to do yourselves good.

5. A Physician is nature's helper, or at least he should be so; whosoever would help nature, must of necessity be well acquainted with her: a little communication between them, will instruct him the way and manner which Almighty God has allotted her to govern the world by; wisdom instructs her Children in the knowledge of time; for there is an appointed time for everything under the Sun: if then when a disease seems extremely dangerous, you would make an essay to relieve languishing nature, do it at the time when the Moon passeth by the body, or good aspect of Jupiter or Venus; then

is nature in a capability of receiving help; you may better lift up a living man with one finger, than a dead man with both hands; a Bird whilst she has wings can fly; but cut off her wings, and hang a couple of Millstones on her legs, she cannot: Even so the bodies, and good aspects of Jupiter and Venus are like wings to carry a man from sickness to health.

6. The bodies and aspects of Saturn and Mars, are like Millstones to weigh him to his Grave.

7. One thing more let me tell you, and I'll tell you but the truth; they say if Saturn afflict, Jupiter helps more than Venus; but if Mars afflict, Venus helps more than Jupiter; let them say so still; but if you will be ruled by me, make use of that fortune which is strongest; a rich friend may relieve your wants; a poor friend cannot, he may wish you well and so forth: but suppose you dare not stay while the Moon come to the good aspect of Jupiter and Venus, administer you medicine when she is in the place, where one of them was at the Decumbiture, if you dare not stay that time neither, for delay is dangerous in acute diseases, be sure you place one of them two in the ascendent, when you administer the medicine; put all these together, and it will tell you in words at length and not in figures that a Physician without Astrology, is like a pudding without fat.

8. That place and state of the Planet, from which the Moon is separated at the Decumbiture, and the condition of the Planet also (for Planets are of different conditions as well as men, some good, and some bad) is to be heeded.

9. If you please to observe the state of that same Planet, by it you may know the state of the sick, and what the cause of his sickness is.

10. When you have done so, it is your wisest way to consider to what Planet the Moon applies; and then do but so much as view what sign that Planet is in, what his conditions be, whether he be benevolent or malevolent; whether he be Masculine or Feminine, Diurnal or Nocturnal, hot, dry, cold or moist; what parts of the body he governs, and what disease he governs.

11. Consider whether the Planet the Moon applies to be in an Angle, in a succeeding, or in a Cadent house; and when you have done so, do but so much as consider what the House he is in signifies; and what members of the body it governs; and then take but a little notice whether the Planet joy in the House or not, that you may not be mistaken herein. I will certify you in what houses every Planet takes his delight, as being confident even amongst Astrologers, more are ignorant of it than know it.

- The Sun rejoices in the fourth, ninth, and eleventh houses.

- The Moon rejoices in the third and seventh houses.

- Saturn rejoices in the ascendent eighth and twelfth houses.

- Jupiter rejoices in the second, ninth, and eleventh.

- Mars rejoices in the third, sixth, and tenth.

- Venus rejoices in the fifth and twelfth,

- Mercury rejoices in the ascendent and sixth. Here's but a few words, yet so significant, that the nature and condition, the Sympathy and Antipathy of the Planets, and by consequence of the Creation, may be known from it: 'Tis not my present scope to tell you which way; whet your wits upon it, and they will be the sharper.

- Consider whether the Planet the moon applies to, be direct or retrograde; swift or slow, in motion, Oriental, Occidental, or Combust, whether fortunated or infortunated by other Planets; and—

- And when you have done so, it is your wisest way to consider whether the threatening Planet be in his own House or Exaltation, or other essential dignities, whether he be in Terms of good Planets or ill; for if a good Planet have gotten an ill Planet in his Term, he will order him. To wind up this in one word, consider whether the threatening Planet has power to execute his will or not; for sometimes a cursed Cow has but short horns.

- Do but so much as note what configurations the Lord of the ascendent, sixth, and eighth Houses have one with another: and amongst the rest, do not forget the lord of the seventh and twelfth Houses, and I'll give you my reason why: the seventh, because it opposes the ascendent; he assaults life openly, and is not ashamed of what he does; he plays the part of Ajax, goes to't with downright blows without policy. The sixth, eighth, and twelfth Houses, have no affinity at all with the ascendent: And they have more of Ulysses in them than Ajax; they take away a man's life when he's asleep, or else when he knows not how.

- Partile aspects are far more strong and prevalent than Platic.

- Be pleased but to consider that the sixth House and his Lord signifies the sickness: the seventh the Physician; the eighth Death; the tenth the Medicine; the fourth, the end of the Disease: and when you have done so, I have done with this point.

These things thus premised, when you have read them, you shall find I first come to —

General Prognostications of the Disease.

1. First of all (quoth my Author) The House of Heaven is of more force than the Sign; and it's very like; and the sign than the Planet; and the Planet than the fixed star he is with: But Doctor Reason told me, the Planet was of more force than the sign, because he was nearer to the earth.

2. If the ascendent, and the luminaries, and their Lords be afflicted by the Malevolent, or by an ill House, or by the Lord of Death, (it's no great matter what star it is) and the benevolents lend no aid, 'tis shrewdly to be suspected the sickness drags death at its tail; he's a wise Physician that can cut the cord.

3. If the forenamed signifiers be well disposed and not afflicted, the fear of death is more than the harm.

4. A Benevolent Planet in the sixth, cures the disease without the help of a Physician.

5. A Malevolent Planet there causes a change in the disease, and usually from better to worse.

6. An infortune in the seventh shows but a paltry Physician, though he be a Collegiate. A fortune there, the contrary.

7. A fortune in the tenth shows proper Physic who ever gives it.

8. A fortune in the fourth brings the disease to a good and speedy end (unless he be Lord of the eight). Every man must do his office; and as the case may be ordered, Jupiter may kill a man as soon as Saturn.

9. Jupiter helps most in cold diseases, Venus in hot.

10. The bodies of Jupiter and Venus soon cure the sick; their Trines and Sextiles will not be much behind hand in the business: And to tell you my own opinion without any complements: the Quartile and Opposition of Jupiter and Venus is better than the Sextile and Trine of Saturn or Mars in this case, unless they be Lord of the ascendent. And by the time you have been acquainted with Dr. Experience but half so long as I have been, he'll make you believe that what I say is true.

11. A Malevolent in the ascendent threatens death; and makes the sick as cross-grained as Bajazet the Turkish Emperor when he was in the iron Cage.

12. Good stars in bad places afflict the humor they govern; they do the like if they be afflicted with malevolent. Was never any of you that reads these lines abused by honest people?

13. The conjunction of the Moon and Mercury is as constant as a weather-cock: the disposition of Mercury is very various according to his position and aspect: With the Fortunes he is better than either. He's just like the people of this Nation; he follows the swing of the times.

14. The Moon in conjunction with the Sun upon a critical day, always portends mischief; and take this for a Maxim from me, and say I told you of it: no aspect is so propitious to the Moon as the Trine and Sextile of the Sun. Nothing so hateful to the squeamish Virgin as hls Conjunction Quartile and Opposition.

15. If the Moon upon a Critical day apply to a malevolent, you'll say that is but a scurvy sign: I am half of your opinion; yet it is good to be wise, and that you may be so, see which of them is strongest, the Moon, or the Malevolent; if the Moon be strongest, she'll make a handsome shift with him: if she be weakest, you know the old Proverb, the weakest goes to the walls, and the sick is like to be forced to make use of a winding-sheet instead of a featherbed.

16. If the Moon upon a Critical day be with the bodies of Sol, Mars, or Saturn; and which of them she's withall, be Lord of the eighth House: away trots life to seek a new habitation; for she's weary of her old House.

17. If the Moon on a Critical day be strong in her House or exaltation, though aspected to no Planet at all; she'll play her part stoutly (for all she is a woman) that she'll restore the sick to his pristine health, if she were not too too much afflicted at the Decumbiture.

18. If the Moon be not at all afflicted at the Decumbiture (as such a thing may be) yet if she be afflicted on the Critical day, a good Crisis cannot be expected: sickness keeps his old house, unless death dispossess him. This in general; but he that would go the wisest way to work in the judging of diseases, must come to particulars. The thing I promised you in this Chapter was gene-

ral Prognostications of diseases, which that I may make lucidly appear to you, (for you shall not find one of Pharaoh's Taskmasters of me, to set you to make Bricks and give you no straw). Be but pleased seriously to weigh in the balance of Reason, these particulars.

- First of all, what diseases every Planet of himself distinctly causes.

- What diseases distinctly are under every several signs of the zodiac.

- What particular part and member of the body every Planet generally rules.

- What particular part and member of the body is under the influence of every sign of the zodiac, and house of the heavens in a Celestial Scheme.

- What part of the body every Planet particularly rules, according to his transit through each sign.

Of all these in Order, and in the same Order they are set down; and if I should happen to be a little critical against my Author, who can help it?

Part I: The diseases the Planets signify.

1. The Sun causes Pimples and Burles in the face, afflictions of the heart; Heartburning, Tremblings, Faintings, Timpanies, sore Eyes, and diseases of the mouth; Cramps, Convulsions, all diseases of the Heart and Brain, and their ascendents, viz. the Nerves and Arteries, Stinking-breath, Catarrhs, rotten fevers; thus Authors. And if any ask why I mention no more, tell them here's more than is true. Now to the purpose.

2. First, of all Timpanies that are under the Moon, I have known the Sun give a fiery disease, but never a watery.

3. Cramps and Convulsions are under the Moon; and so are all diseases that often return, as Agues do: you shall find the same in another Aphorism afterwards; and although my Author contradict himself, I do not delight to imitate him in that sport.

4. The Head, Brain, and Nerves, are not under the Sun, as you shall hear hereafter.

5. Catarrhs are under either Mercury or Jupiter, or both; take this for a Maxim of truth, and say I told you so. A Planet ruling a part of the body, if he be weak in the Genesis, that part of the body is naturally weak: I confess I know not wherefore Art was made, unless to help nature. The eyes are under the Luminaries, and whosoever has them weak in their Genesis, has but weak fight. The Lungs are under Jupiter; Mercury is the opposite Planet to Jupiter. Now then, if Jupiter be weak, he is not able to strengthen the Lungs as he should do; if Mercury be the afflicting Planet, he weakens the Lungs by opposition. If you have but wit enough to know by a penny how a shilling's coined,

6. Sensibus hecimis imis (res non & parva) repone.

7. Afford these lines a place amidst your senses,

8. And be not gulled by specious pretenses.

9. I have now leaped from the Sun to the Moon, and she (they say) causes Apoplexies, Palsies, Cholic, Belly-ache, diseases in the Stones, Bladder, and instruments of Generation; stopping and overflowing of the Terms in Women, Dropsies, Fluxes, all cold and Rheumatic diseases, Gout, Sciatica, Worms in the Belly, Rhumes [colds], and hurts in the Eyes; Surfeits, rotten Coughs, Convulsions, Falling-sickness, King's-Evil, Apostumes, small Pox, and Measles; all coagulated and crude humors

in any part of the body, Lethargies, and all diseases of Phlegm; thus my Author.

10. Amongst these I except against,

- Apoplexies, and you shall find my reason within a quarter of an hour, unless you fall asleep with reading.

- Diseases in the Instruments of Generation, for they are caused by Venus and Mars; by the one by Sympathy, by the other by Antipathy.

- The Gout is caused by Saturn. Who knows but that's the reason why he moves so slowly?

11. Now must I leave the Moon, and mount up to Saturn, for I am like the World, never in a Station.

12. Under Saturn, say Authors, are Apoplexies, Toothache, Quartain Agues; all diseases which come of Melancholy, cold and dryness. Leprosy, Rhumes, Consumptions, Black-Jaundice, Palsies, Trembling, vain-fears, formidable fancies of a Hobgoblin, Dropsies, Gouts of all sorts; a Dog-like-hunger, Hemorrhoids, broken Bones, and Dislocations, Deafness, pain in the bones, Ruptures if he be in Leo or Scorpion, or in an ill aspect to Venus: Iliac passion, Chin-cough, Catarrhs, pains in the Bladder, all long diseases, all madness that comes of Melancholy, fear or grief.

13. If you will give me leave (after I have been first a little Critical) I will be (secondly) a little instructive.

14. nested I except against Apoplexies; and if you would learn why; you shall so soon as you have learned a little Patience.

15. I except against Dropsies, for they are under the Moon.

16. I except against Catarrhs, for they are under Jupiter or Mercury, or both.

17. I except against Dog-like hunger, for it's under Mars.

- A few instructions would I very willingly give you, if I thought you would be so wise to heed them. I had as good give them you under Saturn, as under another Planet. I will not give them to you under each Planet, because he's a foolish Musician that harps always on one string.

- A planet causes diseases.

- By Sympathy.

- By Antipathy.

18. And as the cause is so must the cure be, unless you will do as Scogging did, strike him that stands next you, because another another abuses you.

19. These diseases Saturn causes by Sympathy: Toothache, broken bones; the reason is because he rules the bones. Deafness he causes because he rules the ears. Melancholy and all diseases of the spleen by the same argument.

20. Second, also he afflicts all the parts of the body that are under the Moon by antipathy; and likewise he plays the same tricks with those that are under the Sun; you shall know what they are by and by. The great wisdom of a Physician is to know whether Saturn cause the disease by Sympathy or Antipathy, and then take nothing, that as the cause is so is the cure, Sympathetical, or antipathetical; and withall do not forget, that sympathetical cures strengthen nature; antipathetical cures, in one degree or another, weaken it: And now your own mother-wit (if you have any) will teach you, that antipathetical Medicines are not to be used,

unless to such patients whom Doctor Ignorance, or Doctor Carelessness, has had so long in hand, that sympathetical will not serve the turn. To bring all this to the point in hand that so it may be useful: If Saturn cause the disease by sympathy, cure it by the sympathetical herbs of Saturn. If he cause the disease by antipathy, note whether it be antipathy to Sun or moon; or if it happen in the instruments of generation, be sure it is by antipathy to Venus. Make use of the sympathetical herbs of those Planets respectively for cure: you shall not live the age of a little fish, before I give you rational instructions for them all, I now leave Saturn and come a little lower to —

21. Jupiter. Jupiter they say causes Apoplexies, all infirmities of the Liver and Veins, inflammations of the Lungs, Plurifies and other Apostumes about the Breast and Ribs, all diseases proceeding of putrefaction of blood and wind, quinsies, fevers, and other diseases; which Authors either for want of witt, or super-abundance of ignorance are pleased to attribute to him.

22. Against these I except:

- Against Apoplexies; for it cannot come about that all the Planets should cause Apoplexies; if so, they would be more frequent than they are.

- Against corruption of blood: For Saturn corrupts the blood by melancholy, and Mars by choler.

23. Mars. Diseases under Mars are pestilences, burning fevers, tertian and quotidian agues, megrim, carbuncles and plague sores; burning, scalding, ring-worms, blisters, frenzy, fury, hare-brains, sudden distempers in the head coming of heat: yellow-jaundice, bloody-flux, fistulas, all

wounds whatsoever. Diseases in the instruments of generation: the stone in the reines and bladder, scars and pock-holes in the face, all hurts by iron and fire, the shingles, falling sickness, calentures, St. Anthony's fire; all diseases coming of choler, anger, or passion.

24. Amongst all these I can justly except but against one; and that is the falling sickness, which is under the Moon. And your self will be of my opinion, if you please but to take notice that those hideous fits usually come at conjunction, opposition and quartile of the Moon to the Sun.

25. Venus. Diseases under Venus are all diseases of the womb whatsoever, as suffocation, precipitation, dislocation, etc. All diseases incident to the members of generation, the reines and navel, as the running of the reines, the French pox, etc. All diseases coming by inordinate love or lust, priapism, impotence in the act of generation, ruptures of all sorts: all diseases belonging to the urine, as dysuria, iscuria and stranguria, iliac passion, diabetes, etc.

26. Against these I except

- Impotence in the act of generation, for that's under Saturn.

- Ruptures, for he has a share in them also.

- Diseases of the urine, for they are under Mars.

- The Iliac passion, which is under Mercury.

27. Mercury. Under Mercury are almost all the diseases of the brain, as vertigo, madness, etc., all diseases of the lungs, as Asthma, Phthisics, etc., all imperfections of the Tongue, as stammering, lisping, etc., Hoarseness, coughs, snuffling in the nose: all defects of the memory, gout, stopping of the head, dumbness, folly and simplicity (the

Epidemical diseases of the time) and whatsoever hurts the intellectual faculty.

28. Against these I except

- Against the defects of the memory, for Saturn has a great share in that.

- Against the Gout for Saturn wholly rules that.

I have now done with this part, and if any youngsters ask why I have not given a Reason for all I have spoken: Tell them the Reason is clear in the matter, and he that is not able to see it, is as unfit to give Physic. A blind man cannot see the Sun on a clear day when he is upon the Meridian.

Part II: What diseases distinctly are under every sign of the zodiac.

1. Under Aries are all pushes, whelks and pimples, freckles and Sun-burning in the face; the small pox and measles, polyps or *noli me tangere*; all diseases in the head, as headache of all sorts; vertigo, frenzy, lethargy, forgetfulness, catalepsy, apoplexy, dead palsy, coma, falling sickness, convulsions, cramps, madness, melancholy, trembling.

2. Amongst all these I can justly except but against one, which is smallpox and measles.

3. Under Taurus all diseases incident to the throat, as King's evil, quinsy, sore throat, wenns in the neck, flux of rheum in the throat.

4. Diseases under Gemini are all such as are incident to the hands, arms and shoulders, whether they come really or by accident, as fractures, dislocations, and such as come by blood-letting, corruption of the blood, windiness in the blood; and indeed I have often found by experience, that Gemini signifies wind in the blood more than any other sign. I have now done with Gemini, after I

have told you my own opinion, which is, that the upper part of the shoulder, namely that with which we carry burdens, is under Taurus, which is the Emblem of labor, and not under Gemini, as the common received opinion is.

5. Under Cancer are all imperfections of the breast, stomach, or liver whatsoever, as also whatsoever are incident to the breasts of women, as Cancers there, and that inflammation, which women commonly call the imposthumes, plurifies, want of appetite to victuals, want of digestion of Victuals, coldness and over-heat of the stomach, dropsies, coughs; you may find out the rest your selves; the rule is as plain as the nose in a man's face.

6. Under Leo are all passions of the heart, as convulsions says my Author.

7. But if I may make so bold as to digress a little, I shall tell you, and prove it too when I have done, that convulsions are not a disease of the heart, but of the brain. The truth is, it is one of old Aristotle's opinions, which crept into his noddle, as he was marring Plato's Philosophy. The nerves have their origin from the brain; convulsion is a plucking, or twitching, of the nerves; ergo it is a disease of the brain and not of the heart.

8. But to return to my purpose; under Leo, are all diseases the heart or back is subject to, as qualms and passions, palpitation, and trembling of the heart, violent burning fevers, sore eyes, the yellow jaundice, and all diseases of choler, and such diseases as come of adustion of blood as the pestilence; and I am afraid London will find this too true so soon as Saturn comes into Leo. I pray God mitigate this evil influence toward them at that time.

9. Under Virgo are all diseases incident to the bowels, the meseraic veins, the omentum, the diaphragm, spleen. Take a few instances in this particular; worms wind in the guts, obstructions, the cholic and iliac, passions, hardness of the spleen, hypochondriac melancholy.

10. Under Libra are diseases of the reines or kidneys, which you please; for the significations of the word are the same; heat of the reines in women, which sometimes causes death in travail, many times abortion, always hard labor; the stone or gravel in the reines. And now let me teach you a little, if Mars be signifier of the disease, and in Virgo, it is the wind-cholic, without appearance either of gravel or stone.

11. Have a care of your patient, lest it turn to gravel in the kidneys when he comes into Libra, and to

12. the stone of the bladder when he comes into the Scorpion.

13. Your own ingenuity, if you have any; you may by this example find out twenty more like to it.

14. Lastly under Libra are all diseases coming of wind and corruptions of blood.

15. Under the Scorpion are gravel and stone in the bladder, inflammations and ulcers there, all difficulties of urine whatsoever; all imperfections of the urine, ruptures, fistulas, hemorrhoids, the French pox, running of the reines, priapism; all diseases that infect the privities of men or women.

16. All diseases of the womb, of which more for my Guide for women already in print.

17. Under Sagittarius are all diseases in thighs and hip; as the Sciatica etc., fistulas in those places, heat of blood, pestilential fevers; and take this for a general rule, that Leo and Sagittarius signifies

fall from horses and hurts by four-footed beasts; they being both of them signs of horsemanship; besides Sagittarius prejudices the body by choler, heat, fire, and intemperance in sports.

18. Under Capricorn are all diseases in the knees and hams; as pains, sprains, fractures, and dislocations, leprosies, itch, scabs, all diseases of melancholy, and all tumors called Schirrus.

19. Under Aquarius are all diseases incident to the Legs and Ankles; all melancholy coagulated in the blood, cramps; and the truth is, thickness of blood most usually proceeds from this sign. Ask old Saturn and he will tell you the reason. By this the ingenuous have a plain way to find out more; and by this Doctor Experience got materials to work with.

20. Under Pisces is all lameness, aches, and diseases incident to the feet, as gouts, kibes, chilblains, etc. All diseases coming of salt phlegm, mixed humors, scabs, itch, botches, and breakings out about the body, the smallpox and measles; all cold and moist diseases, and such as come by catching wet and cold at the feet.

21. And if you will be pleased but to consider the affinity Pisces holds with Aries, you will soon see a reason why wet taken at the feet strikes so speedily up to the head.

22. As for the houses of the heavens, they have the same significations with the signs; the first house with Aries, the second with Taurus, and so analogically till you come to the twelfth house, which has the same significations that Pisces has.

I have now done with this part, only be pleased to take notice that the fiery signs stir up diseases of choler; airy signs, diseases of blood and wind; earthly signs diseases of melancholy; watery signs diseases of phlegm; signs of double bodies, diseases of mixed humors.

And thus much for this part, the pains of which have been mine, the benefit shall be yours; if you will turn but idleness out of Doors, and place ingenuity in his room.

Part III: The particular parts and Members of the body, which the Planets generally rule.

Herein I must either be a little critical, or else part from my loving friend Doctor Reason: I am loathe to do the latter, and therefore must make bold with the former.

1. Saturn, say Authors, rules in the body of man the Spleen, and there he keeps his Court; the right Ear, the Bladder, the Bones, the Breech, the retentive faculties throughout the body; which what it is, be pleased to see my short Treatise of human virtues, in the latter of my Ephemerides, for Anno 1651 where you shall find not only what it is, but also what it is good for.

2. Against all this I except but against only one, which is the Bladder, for that is under the dominion of the Moon.

3. They say Jupiter rules the Lungs, Ribbs, Sides, Liver, Veines, Blood, the digestive faculty, the natural virtue of man which he rules, as Lawyers call it, toto & in solid.

4. Besides, Authors say, he rules the Arteries and Seed; but how they can bring it about I know not, nor I think themselves neither: why should Jupiter rule the Arteries, when the Sun rules the Heart?

5. He that can give a reason *erit mihi magnus* Apollo, and as little reason can be given, and that's little enough, why Jupiter should rule the Seed, which is dame Venus her fee-simple; surely the Planets will not rob one another, though men do; howsoever

Jupiter seems to keep his Court in the Liver; and if you are minded to strengthen his operations in your bodies, begin there.

6. Mars rules in the body of man, the Gall, the Reines, the Veins, the Secrets, the left Ear; thus Authors; and there are but two true words in it, which is the Gall, and the left Ear. The truth is, he rules the apprehension, and that's the reason that choleric men are so quick-witted.

7. Yea, a man of a mean apprehension when he is angry, will make a quicker apprehension in things satisfying his fury than a man of a quicker apprehension has when he is pleased. Anger summons up all the powers of the body and mind to revenge wrong, though it be but imaginary. And then again, Mars rules that faculty which incites men to valor; he makes a man a Soldier every inch of him; he fortifies the smell; and that's the reason Martical creatures have so good smells, as Dogs etc.

8. But every little reason, or none at all; unless you will make a reason of traditions, who derives his pedigree rather from Dr. Corruption than Doctor Reason: Why, Mars should rule the Veins, seeing Jupiter rules the Liver. If Jupiter rules the fountain, shall he be denied the streams? And then the Reines and Secrets are under Venus, and that's apparent without any more dispute of the story.

9. Venus rules the Womb, the Testicles, Yard, and all the instruments of Generation, the Reines or Kidneys, the Throat, Women's breasts, and the Milk contained within them, the Seed, and Liver.

10. But by my Author's favor, I can give no other reason why Venus should rule the Liver, unless I should give this for a reason: because Jupiter stole

the seed from her before, she to quit scores with him, steals away the Liver from him.

11. Under the dominion of Mercury is the brain, especially the rational part of it; the imagination, the tongue, hands and feet, the motional part of man.

12. And that's the reason Mercuriarists (if Mercury be strong) are so swift in motions, so fluent of speech.

13. He gives a quick apprehension, a strong imagination and conceited; he makes a good Pen-man, and stirs up that faculty in man which causes a thirst after knowledge; he is very fickle in his disposition, and that's that that makes men so fickleheaded.

14. If Saturn vouchsafe him a friendly look, he is very constant; otherwise, if you look upon a Weather-cock, you may safely draw his Picture, and no disparagement to his person neither.

15. The Sun governs, if you will believe Authors, the Brain and Nerves, the Heart and Arteries, the sight, the eyes; and in the eyes, the right eye of a man, the left eye of a woman. Against these I except, against the Brain and Nerves, the bulk of which is under the Moon.

16. Their operation is under Mercury; now then if Mercury afflicts the Brain, the failing is in the operation.

17. If the Moon is in the Bulk or body of the Brain, or Nerves he that is a Physician, knows what the operations of nature are: and then he knows what I say is truth, and the foundation of it built upon a Rock. He will esteem it as a Jewel.

18. It is the property of a Fool to carp at what he cannot imitate.

19. Under the Moon is the Bulk of the brain, the stomach, the bowels, the bladder, the taste, the left

eye of a man, the right eye of a woman: a team of Horses cannot draw one to believe that the moon rules the taste.

20. If you please to peruse my Treatise of humane virtues, at the latter end of my Ephemerides for Anne 1651, I think you shall find there that Jupiter rules it: and my reason for it may there be found. Besides, I have something from Doctor Experience for it, my own taste being exceeding good, and yet the moon exceeding weak in my Genesis.

21. Being in a Cadent House, and in Genesis, a sign which in my opinion more afflicts the moon than Capricorn.

22. I confess Mr. Lilly affirms Gemini to be a most noble sign, but I dare scarce believe him. Aries is the most principal of all the signs; Gemini is cadent from Aries Ergo, etc. But not now to enter into a Contest with that famous man, to whom this Nation is so much beholding.

23. Be pleased to take notice, that the twelfth House is more inimical to the ascendent, than the seventh; which, if so, then is the moon more afflicted in Gemini, than in Capricorn.

Part IV: The particular parts of the body, under the several signs of the zodiac, and the houses in the Heavens in a Celestial Scheme.

1. Under Aries is the head, and whatever belongs to it, as its Bones, the Face, Brain, Hair, Beard, Eyes, Ears, Nose, Tongue, Teeth etc. whatsoever in man is above the first Vertebra of the Neck.

2. Under Taurus is the Neck, Throat, the Vertebrae of the Neck, which are in number seven. The channel bone, the shoulder blade, according to my opinion.

3. Also Taurus has again signification in the voice; for he will roar like a Bull.

4. Under Gemini are the shoulders, shoulder bones, Arms, Hands, Fingers; together with their bag and baggage.

5. Under Cancer is the Breast, Ribs, Lungs, Pleura, the Ventricle of the stomach, women's Breasts, the Liver, Spleen etc. and yet Doctor Reason told me the other night, that the Spleen was under Virgo.

6. Under Leo is the heart, the back, and the Vertebrae of the breast, which are in number twelve; the Pericardium; some Authors say the stomach is under Leo, but I can scarce believe it: I am persuaded the Appetite is under Leo, and that's the reason such as have that sign ascending in their Genesis, are such greedy eaters.

7. You that are Astrologers, and have the Nativity of such persons in your hands, you know my words are truth.

8. And if in a Nativity, the prevalence of other signifiers should happen to contradict it:

9. You know the old proverb, one Swallow makes out a summer.

10. Under Virgo is the Belly and Bowels, the Navel and Spleen, the Omentum, and all their Appurtenances etc.

11. This is that she rules, and she bids you by my pen to be chaste.

12. Under the balance, say Authors, are the Reines, Loins, and Kidneys, between which in my judgment is as much difference as is between eight pence and two groats. Under Libra besides, they say, are the Hams, Buttocks, Bladder, and Navel; thus Authors. And I quoted it only to this end, that young Students may see what a monster tradition is and

may avoid being led by the Nose by it, as Bears are led to the Stake. You know well enough if the blind lead the blind, what will become of them both: Let every one that desires to be called by the name of Artist have his wits in his head, (for that's the place ordained for them) and not in his books.

13. The Hams are under Capricorn, the Bladder under Scorpio, the Navel under Virgo; ask Doctor Reason, and see if he tell you not the same tale.

14. Under Scorpio are the Secrets of both Sexes; it is not very fitting for me to name them; as also the seminal Vessels; all the vessels dedicated to the Generation of man, the bladder and fundament; and therefore though artists cry out so much against the Scorpion for a false, deceitful, treacherous, mischievous, violent, poisonous sign. Let them look back to the rock from whence they are hewn: It may be they shall see the reasons of some of their violent speeches against my self. A word is enough to wise men. Let them not speak evil of what they know not.

15. This is is most certain, from those parts of the body under the dominion of Scorpio have all men and women in general the influence of their propagation;

16. And in them take they their greatest pleasure; and thus have I spoken something for a sign which everyone speaks against.

17. Time will not stay, therefore I must be brief: under Sagittarius are the thighs, the bone called *Os sacrum*, which whether justly so called, or unjustly, I know not. It is either Jewish superstition or worse. The rump-bone, the thigh-bone, together with all the appurtenance belonging to the thigh.

18. Some Authors say the hams are under Sagittarius, but then they are beside the Cushion.

19. Under Capricorn are the knees, hams, and what belongs unto them.

20. Under Aquarius are the legs and whatsoever belongs unto them, even from the outward skin called Cuticula, to the midst of the marrow in both bones; for these are two of them, which Chirurgeons [surgeons], because they would keep you in ignorance, called, *Focile majus* and *Focile minus*, or if you will, tibia and fibula. They all know what the bones are but a quarter of them are not able to give you a reason why the bones are so called. Pray take notice of this in going about to make slaves of you, they have made fools of themselves.

21. Lastly, Pisces claims the feet and ankles, toes and all the bones. To write like a scholar 'tis tarsus metatarsus, and the bones of the toes. It rules also the skin of the foot, the flesh and vessels between the skin and the bones.

22. For though the sign be the weakest in the zodiac, it is unwilling altogether to leave you nought but skin and bones.

23. Also some Authors hold an opinion that the signs carry the same signification in order that the houses of heaven do; and that Aries should signify life; Taurus estate; Gemini Brethren and short journeys; you know the rest. Truly, my own opinion is, many Authors invented whimsies, and when they had done, set them down to posterity for truth; who taking them up without tryall, clothed Tradition in Plush, and left poor reason to go in Rags. An Author said so; ergo 'tis true, right or wrong.

24. I take this to be one of that generation, and I prove it thus; by this account Cancer should rule the Fathers; but experience tells us that an ill Planet in

Cancer in the genesis threatens evil to the Mother, but in Leo to the Father. A word is enough to a wise man.

25. Also there is another signification of the Planets according to the respective signs therein; every Planet making his Aries in his own house. I forbear it here; first of all because it conduces not much to my present scope; for example, a Urine came to me about a year ago; Mercury was the afflicting Planet, and in Aries, according to this rate Mercury rules the legs and privities; but the man was diseased in his head, for he was mad.

26. I gave you a table of it in my Guide for women; and I am as loathe to write one thing twice, as you are to pay for one thing twice. If this will not content you, you are so hard to be pleased that I shall not undertake to please you, but to please myself; and in so doing I am confident to please somebody else.

How the nature and kind of the Disease may be found out by the Figure of the decumbiture.

1. The nature of the disease is found out three ways. First, by the houses of heaven, of which the 6th, 7th, and 12th signify diseases.

2. By the nature of the signs, of which fiery sign signify choler and diseases thence proceeding; earthly signs signify the diseases of melancholy, airy signs diseases of blood and wind; watery signs, diseases of water and salt phlegm.

3. By the Planets themselves and their aspects. All this I shall make clear, by this subsequent

discourse, before which I shall premise these following Aphorisms: 1. If Saturn signifies the disease, 'tis like to continue long enough, if not too long; yet if he be with benevolents it mitigates: if with malevolents it increases the evil. 2. Saturn in Leo, or Capricorn with the Dragon's head or tail, or with Venus combust, or with violent fixed stars, he stirs up pestilences, or other pernicious fevers that are little better. 3. Saturn alone in fiery signs shows Hectic fevers.

4. In watery signs sickness or watery humors. The disease comes of gross and vicious humors, which will continue long with continual fluxes and cold tremblings.

5. Saturn in moveable signs shows flux of humors in all parts of the body. Imagine the Dropsy or other diseases like to it; and yet it is some question to me, whether Saturn cause Dropsies yea or no, unless assisted by the Moon in signification.

6. Saturn in common signs gives compound diseases, and such as run out of one disease into another, and yet they pass leisurely out of one disease into another to, you may almost whip a snail as fast; you may easily see it before it come if your eyes be in your head.

7. Saturn in fixed signs, if in Leo, gives hectic fevers, in other fixed signs quartane agues, gouts, leprosies, and other diseases that stay longer than they are welcome.

8. If Jupiter causes the disease, look to the Liver for that's afflicted, the digestion is bad; blood abounds either in quantity or quality; a thousand to one if it be not too hot.

9. Jupiter in fiery signs bestows upon men such fevers as come of blood without putrefaction, such as the

Greeks call *Synochus non putrida*; they last but a very little while.

10. Mars gives violent fevers with putrefactions, and the Sun gives no other.

11. If you find Mars in a fiery sign, judge the disease either a burning fever called [...], or else the pestilence; if Saturn bear a share in signification with him, melancholy bears a share, or else a dusk choler which is more usual.

12. Mars in common signs varies the disease; take heed of relapse; the Crisis is as certain as a weather-cock, so exceeding swift and sudden will they come, even as swift as the wind not waiting the Moon's leisure. In such a case you may more safely judge by the aspects of the Moon to the Planets than by the Crisis.

13. Mars in Leo afflicts the heart, the disease is a fever, and the cause of it Choler.

14. Always when Mars signifies the disease, it is very short but extremely acute.

15. If the Sun at the decumbiture be afflicted by the body or Quartile Opposition, Antiscion of Saturn, the disease is Saturning Melancholy, and will in all probability last longer than you would willingly have it.

16. If the Sun be afflicted in the same manner by Mars, the cause is choler; the motion of the disease is as swift as the wind, and as violent as the whirlwind.

17. If Venus be ill affected to the sick, the disease comes of Intemperance, either one way or another; perhaps with drinking, perhaps by venereal sports; what ere the cause be, those parts of the body signified by Venus suffer for it.

18. Venus in fiery signs causes one-day fevers; but if Mars joins with her in signification, the fever is rotten and proceeds from phlegm.

19. If Mercury be infortunate and cause the disease, he proclaims that the infirmity lies in the brain, perhaps madness, or falling sickness, or it may be the man dreams waking.

20. If Mercury joins in signification with Mars, you may be confident the disease is a frenzy.

21. The Lord of the ninth in the sixth, witchcraft is to be feared, or else the disease lies very occult; I doubt my Author is mistaken: surely it should be the Lord of the 12th in the 6th, for the Lord of the 9th should rather occasion the disease about some whimsies in Religion.

22. The Moon in Aries in the 8th afflicts the head with a disease too hot for it to bear, whether the disease lie in the mind, or in the body.

How to know whether the disease be in the mind or in the body.

All the Aphorisms of my Author upon this question are got so deeply together by the ears, and in such a hubbub, that I know not in the world which way to go about to reconcile them; every following Aphorism thwarts him that goes before; in one he affirms that the Sun, Moon, and ascendent rule the body, and the Lord the mind; the very next Aphorism affirms the contrary; most of them contradict one another in such a hideous manner, that I was forced to leave their companies and search other Authors for a resolution of this point; and they conclude that the Sun, Moon, and Ascendent signifies the body, and their Lord the mind; and if this may be taken for truth, the directive Aphorisms are these:

1. The Sun, Moon, and Lord of the Ascendent impeded, and their Lord safe shows the disease lies in the body and not in the mind.

2. If their Lord be impeded and they safe, the disease lies in the mind and not in the body.

3. If both Sun, Moon, and the Ascendent and their Lord also be impeded, or the greatest part of them, both body and mind are diseased; and this I confess is something rational.

4. Saturn generally signifies melancholy, and by consequence alienation of mind, madness, etc. and therefore always you find him to be signifier of the disease, or in the ascendent, or in the 6th house afflicting the Lord of the Ascendent, or either of the Luminaries; the sick is afflicted with care or grief or something else that's as bad; be sure the mind suffers for it.

5. If Jupiter be signifier of the disease, it lies in the body, if it lie anywhere; for Jupiter never troubles, unless it be that Monster which men call Religion.

6. It were a good thing when a man is troubled in mind, if an Artist could tell the cause of this, his trouble, that you may do so, make use of these two or three rules; there is enough of them though there be but few, if you have but witt enough to know by a penny how a shilling is coined; they are these:

   - If the Sun be Author of the distemper, as he may be if he be Lord of the House Ascendent 6th or 12th houses; the distemper comes through pride, ambition, or vainglory.

   - If it be Jupiter, it comes through religion, some idle Priest has scar'd the poor creature out of his wits.

- If it be Venus, Love, luxurious expense, or something else of like nature is the cause.

- If Mercury be the afflicting Planet, the sick is pestered with a parcel of strange imaginations, and as many vain fears attend him; great vexation or study, or both is the cause.

By these you may find out all the rest; for this is the sum of the business.

How it may be known what part of the body is afflicted.

That this may be known, for 'tis not only possible, but also probable, be pleased to consider,

1. If the sign the Lord of the 6th possesses, especially if he be an infortune, or a fortune infortunated. And then,

2. Consider what part of the body the sign he is in governs, as Aries governs the head, Taurus the neck and throat, etc. and be sure that part's afflicted.

3. Consider what parts of the body the afflicting Planet rules, which are under that sign, and you need not question but that's afflicted.; for example, Venus though she rule many parts of the body, yet in Scorpio she rules under the privities.

4. Saturn Lord of the 6th and in the 10th in Taurus afflicts the body universally, but especially the left side.

5. Saturn Lord of the sixth in the last degrees of Gemini, or in the first degree of Cancer, causes pain in the left side, as though an Awl were running to it.

6. Saturn Lord of the 6th in Leo in the second house causes pains in the back and heart; the original of which says my Author, is blood, but I should rather think it Melancholy.

7. If he be in Virgo, the 12th house signifies pain in the head; if he be in Mars oriental and slow in motion, signifies diseases in the Reines, as the gravel, stone, and pissing blood. I confess I can give no reason for all this.

8. If Saturn be Lord of the disease and in Aquarius, the disease comes by travail.

9. Mars Lord of the 6th and in the 5th and in Scorpio gives an internal pain in all parts of the body; if it be a woman she is not well in her womb, the illness of which afflicts all her body, especially her head, by reason of that admirable congruity betwixt that part and her womb; kind women, take notice of it; for it is as true as that the Sun is up when he is upon the meridian. All Cephalic medicines help the womb and remedy its grief; I am confident you desire a reason of it, you shall not fail of your desires. It is because Aries and Scorpio are both the Houses of Mars.

10. If Mars be retrograde in Scorpio and in the Ascendent, the whole body is universally afflicted, but externally, viz. the man breaks out in boils and ulcers, or itch, perhaps it is the smallpox or measles; if Venus set forward the mischief, the French pox is shrewdly to be suspected.

11. If Mars be Lord of the 6th in Leo, the sick is extremely pained in his back, in this you need never fear failing.

12. If Mars be Lord of the 6th in Virgo, my Author says it will lie in the left side, or left leg. But after I had had half an hour's talk with Dr. Experience,

he proved to me it was always the Colic, and heat in the bowels; take heed it comes not to the gravel in the kidneys, when Mars comes into Libra: and to the stone in the bladder, when Mars comes to Scorpio. He that is a Physician knows as well how to prevent a disease before it comes, as how to remedy it when it is come.

13. The Moon in the Ascendent afflicted by Saturn or Mars, bestows difficulty of breathing, and infirmities in the lungs upon a man; I confess I can give no reason for it.

14. Venus, Lady of the 6th and infortunated by Mars, gives suspicions enough in the French pox.

15. Here is enough to teach you more; let not all your wits lie in your books; be diligent and studious, or else you may happen to die fools; let not all your wits lie in your books, but some in your heads; it is within you, and not that without you must do you good.

As for the side of the body afflicted, my Author has left a few rules to know it, which I will declare to you, and leave them to the approbation or exprobration of Dr. Experience; they are these,

1. If the Lord of the sixth house be afflicted above the earth, and in a diurnal sign, the sickness is in the right side of the body, and in the upper part of it.

2. If the Lord of the 6th be under the earth, and in a nocturnal sign, the sickness lies in the inferior parts of the body, and on the left side.

3. Whether he be under or above the earth in a diurnal, the sickness is in the forepart of the body, imagine the forehead, face, breast, belly, or some other visible part.

4. If it be in a nocturnal sign, the disease lies in the back parts of the body, or else in some part but lies invisible, as the bowels, etc., or perhaps the disease lies occult; for take this for a general rule, the diseases are more hidden from the eyes of your understanding, when the signifiers of them are in nocturnal signs than they are when they are in Diurnal.

5. If the signifiers be corrupted by other Planets, and a difference in these rules between the signifier and the planet that corrupts them, the patient is afflicted both ways; namely according as he signifies, and according as the Planet corrupting signifies.

6. In such a case, view diligently which of them is most afflicted: and your reason, if you have any, will tell you, that the most part of the malady lies in that part of the body signified by the Planet which is most afflicted.

7. To wind up all in a word: Masculine Planets denote the right side of the body, Feminine the left, all of them afflict that part of the body which they govern.

Whether the disease shall be long or short, or whether it shall end in Life or Death.

For judging of this, take a few cautions by the way.

1. Consider if the Sun, Moon, Ascendent and their Lords be much or little afflicted.

2. Consider the age of the sick party; for old age brings longer sickness than youth.

3. Consider the time of the year; for Autumn and Winter bring longer sickness than Spring or Summer.

4. Consider the complexion of the Patient; for a melancholy man is more subject to retain a sickness than a choleric.

5. Consider the Planet afflicting; for Saturn produces longer sickness than Mars.

6. The Planets generally and briefly order the sickness they give in this manner; Saturn gives long sickness, the Sun in Jupiter short, Mars shorter than either of them, but acute; Venus mean; Mercury various and unconstant, according to the Planet he is joined with or aspected. The Moon gives such sickness as often return, as Agues, falling sickness, etc. And, therefore, the direction of the Moon to the body, or in aspect to Saturn will sooner cause a falling sickness than the direction of any other signifier.

These are the cautions, and according to these cautions so understand these following Aphorisms, which you shall find marshaled into these three divisions: First, Signs of long or short sickness. Secondly, signs of recovery. Thirdly, signs of death.

Part I: Signs of long or short sickness.

1. First, the 6th house being possessed by a fixed sign, argues length in the disease; if the sign that possesses the Cusp by the 6th be moveable, the disease will be short; if the sign be common, the disease will either be mean in respect of length, or else a change of the disease, or a relapse is to be feared.

2. If the latter degrees of a sign be upon the Cusp of the 6th, the disease will quickly end either one way or another.

3. A fixed sign under Cusp of the 6th shows tough and hard humors to be the causes of the disease, and such as are hard to be expelled, they stick to the body like birdlime.

4. Saturn Lord of the 6th shows long diseases; Jupiter, Mars and the Sun short; Mercury such as are as constant as the weathercock.

5. If the Lord of the 6th be stronger than the Lord of the Ascendent, the sickness gets strength against nature: if you find it so upon a figure in urine, judge the disease increases.

6. If the Lord of the 6th be weaker than the Lord of the ascendent, nature gets strength over the disease and will at last put him to a total rout.

7. Common signs show the disease will stay in one state, as long as a Cat is tied to a Pudding.

8. The Lord of the 6th, if he be a Malevolent, it is an ill omen; if he be a benevolent, you need not so much as fear a long sickness; for the disease will be cured both speedily and easily, unless the said benevolent be Lord also of the 8th.

9. If the Moon applies to the Lord of the 6th, the disease will be increased till it has put life to its trumps.

10. If the moon be Lady of the ascendent, ill diet was the cause of it; perhaps a surfeit by drinking.

11. If Venus be Lady of the 6th, 'tis women, or it may be sports and pastimes, or such gewgaws as Venus delights in: you know how to judge the rest of the Planets according to their several natures.

12. If the Lord of the sixth applies to the Quartile or Opposition of the Lord of the ascendent, the disease increases, and has not yet come to his height.

13. I confess this, and many other Aphorisms hereabouts, belong not at all to the Decumbitures; but to questions upon Urine, and most of them, if not all of them, will hold true in them also.

14. The Lord of the 6th and 8th is but a scurvy unlucky sign, and shows the sickness will end in death: if it be in the 4th, it shows the sickness will end in the Grave.

15. The Lord of the 6th and the 12th cries aloud that the Patient opposes his own health.

16. The Lord of the 8th in the 6th and the Lord of the 6th in the 8th; if they be in friendly aspect, the sick soon recovers.

17. I confess the former Aphorism seems a paradox to me; I should rather think sickness and death had made a match together, to take away the life of the Patient, and shall do so still, till I have spoken with Doctor Experience about it.

18. If there be an Opposition, Sextile, or Trine between the Lord of the sixth and Jupiter, the sick soon recovers; for Jupiter will handle him without mittens, and 'tis very probable Venus will not come much behind them in the business.

19. Even in such a case Jupiter be in the ninth House, the sickness comes by reason of some Physic formerly taken, which will at last much conduce to the Patient's health.

20. I doubt my Author mistook the ninth House for the tenth; did I say I doubted it? Nay, I know it.

21. It is the tenth house, that it is, the house of Physic, and not the ninth.

22. A malevolent in the 6th is an ill sign; but a benevolent there is as good a one for all that.

23. The Lord of the 12th, and the 6th shows Witch-craft, or possession by the Devil, that's as bad: and if he be a malevolent, you may take it for granted, 'tis as sure as a club.

24. The Lord of the ascendent in the 6th and the Lord of the 6th in the ascendent, show long diseases; and such as will continue till one of them, if not till both of them make his exit out of the sign he is in.

25. If in such a case the malevolent cast ill aspect to her, bid her Physician use his wits as far as he can, though the fear of death is not small.

26. The Lord of the Ascendent and 6th house, in Quartile, Opposition, or Conjunction, in such degrees as Artists call Azemini, and in Angles, threatens such perpetual pain, which none but Doctor Death is likely to cure.

27. The Lord of the 6th in the ascendent, shows the disease will continue long enough, nay longer then 'tis welcome; but it does not signifY the sick must needs die; for that belongs to the 8th house and his Lord.

28. 'Tis no good sign of quick recovery, when the Lord of the 6th house is a malevolent.

29. If the Sun, Moon, and Lord of the ascendent be free from ill beams of ill Planets, and apply to fortunes that are anything strong and like to do good, the cure will come as soon as you can in reason hope for it.

30. 'Tis always bad when the Sun, moon, or Lord of the ascendent apply to the Lord of 6th, 8th, or 12th houses; and 'tis not a whit better, if they be Lord of those houses.

31. It is an exceedingly good sign at the beginning of a sickness, if neither the Lord of the ascendent, Sun nor Moon behold the Lord of the 6th or 8th houses.

32. It's very ill when the Lord of the ascendent is afflicted, namely if he be retrograde or in an ill house, in his detriment or fall, or besieged the malevolents. All houses which behold not the ascendents are ill houses; namely the 6th, 8th, and 12th. I will take no notice at all of the second in this case, because it is succeeding to the first; but the 7th shall not escape so, because it opposes the ascendents: it is very bad when the Lord of the ascendent is there.

33. In such cases, 'tis true the disease may happily be cured, if good courses be taken; but either a relapse into that disease is to be feared, or else the disease is subject to a change out of that disease into another as bad, whereby the sick is in danger of death, unless the mean season the Lord of the ascendent grows stronger; for the stronger he is, the better able he is to preserve life.

34. The Lord of the ascendent infortunated by the Lord of the 6th though he be but in his term, prolongs the sickness.

35. If the Lord of the ascendent be infortunated by the lord of the 8th gives fear enough, that none but death can end the quarrel between the sick and the sickness.

36. If the lord of the ascendent be slow in motion, the sickness will be as slow in the parting, and slower if Saturn be lord of the ascendent: but if the lord of the ascendent be swift in motion, according to the haste he makes, such speed you may expect of the disease.

37. The lord of the ascendent angular and strong, and no way impeded, let the disease be never so violent, the fear of death is more than the harm.

38. The lord of the ascendent entering into another sign, though it be out of his own house into another; provided it be not into the house of the lord of the 6th, 8th or 12th, the disease soon ends in health; if it be into the house of the lord of the 8th, the sick dies at the time; if it be into the house of the lord of the 6th, the sickness is increased; if into the house of the lord of the twelfth, the sick either keeps ill diet, or is unruly, or is mad to take supper in another word; in such a case, he that will not be ruled by reason, must be ruled by force.

39. If the lord of the ascendent be weak of himself, yet if he joined to a fortune, the recovery will be very speedily; for if the fortune be anything strong, he will help it forward with tooth and nail.

40. The lord of the ascendent, the Sun, or the moon joined to an infortune, prolongs the disease; and the weaker they are, the longer is the disease like to last.

41. If the signifier of the disease be in a sign of the nature of the disease: for example, suppose the disease proceeds of melancholy, if the signifier be in an earthly sign, it exceedingly prolongs the disease; judge the like by the rest of the humors; in such cases the cure is exceeding difficult; *vis unita fortior.*

42. If the signifier of the sickness be an infortune, and applied to the lord of the ascendent, it mightily retards the cure; you see what need there is the Physician be an Astrologer; I know not how a man should help nature, unless he knows it.

43. If the moon be with the lord of the ascendent, or applied to him, the cure comes gallantly on, if she be swift in motion; but if she be slow in motion, she hails the cure back-wards.

44. If the moon decrease both in light and motion, and be with the Quartile, Opposition, or body of Saturn, the disease is extreme; for the next time she comes to his body or opposition, unless you can cure the disease before, and he is a Physician indeed that can do it, death takes possession of the breathless Corpse of the Patient.

45. The moon, or any other signifier of the sick joined to a Planet direct and swift in motion, shows but a short sickness; but if the Planet be retrograde or slow, the cure will be as slow to a hair.

46. If Scorpion ascends, the sick is the causer of his own sickness; because then Aries is upon the cusp of the 6th house and one Planet is lord of both places; and if he be in either of both those houses, it is so much the worse, for he will add fire to the fuel, and blow the Bellows too.

47. Both the Luminaries in Cadent houses and their dispositors together with the lord of the ascendent afflicted, shows a disease so dangerous that the Physician has need enough to look about him.

48. If in such a case the benevolents set the helping hands, the disease will be prolonged, and ever acute become chronic; yet if the benevolent be strongest, the disease will at last be cured beyond all hope; if the malevolents be strongest, 'tis shrewdly to be feared, that death must turn Physician when all comes to all.

49. Suppose Mars be lord of the ascendent, and in the 6th yet if he be in any aspect to Venus, 'tis not desperately bad, because she mitigates his evil.

50. The lord of the 6th in the 8th afflicted by Saturn or Mars, if he be weak, viz. retrograde or combust, or in his detriment, the disease will continue till death cures it.

51. The Sun, Moon, or lord of the ascendent with a fortune, and that fortune they are with retrograde, promises cure; but together with the promise, comes a threatening of length of the disease.

52. The Moon in a blad place of the heavens, prolongs the disease if she be in a fixed sign, without any further dispute of the story.

53. Never forget this general rule, the stronger the Moon is at the decumbiture, the better it is for the sick; the weaker she is at that time, the worse.

54. It were a good thing and very commendable if the nativity of the sick could be procured; for if Saturn be Lord of the Nativity, the sick may live, though the Moon be in with his body, or opposition at the decumbiture.

55. Judge of the length or shortness of the disease according as the disease is; for it is not to be expected that a fever should last seven years; and it is as little to be hoped that a Consumption should be cured in a day.

Part 2: Signs of life at the Decumbiture.

1. First, Jupiter, Venus, the Sun and Moon in the Ascendent, not afflicting nor beholding the Lord of the 8th, nor being Lord of the 8th themselves, take away not onely the fear of death, but also promise a speedy cure.

2. The conjunction of the Moon with Jupiter is always prosperous; most propitious if it be in Cancer; if doubtful at all, it is when they are in Capricorn, because in the one they are both dignified; in the

other both Cadent from their dignities; And yet let me tell you but this much, Jupiter is Jupiter still, be he where he will.

3.   The Moon in an angle well disposed in good terms, and free from the body in [...] beams of Saturn or Mars, it restores the sick to health, and scorns to be beholding to any of them all.

4.   The Moon applying to the Lord of the Ascendent, unless she carries the beams of the Lord of death to him, does the like.

5.   The Moon increasing in light and swift in motion, and not posited in the 6th, 8th, nor 12th houses; applying to the Sextile, Trine, or antiscion of Lord of the Ascendent, though the Lord of the ascendent be a malevolent, it matters not, so he be direct, and not infortuned by house, nor impedited by another malevolent, neither in his detriment nor fall; it promises recovery.

6.   If the Moon be void of course at the decumbiture, if on the Critical day she beholds a good star, there is no question of recovery to be made.

7.   If on a Critical day the Moon be in her own house or exaltation, though she be void of course, the fear of death is more than the harm; for the sick will recover.

8.   The Sun, Moon, and Lord of the Ascendent free from the beams of Saturn, Mars, or the Lord of death at the Decumbiture, there cannot be so much as a bare suspicion of death.

9.   If the benevolence be stronger than the malevolence at the decumbiture, and withall if they behold the Moon the Ascendent or his Lord, they promise recovery. The Malevolence may threaten hard etc., but the benevolence will stay the deadly blow.

10. If the Moon be separated from a weak malevolent, and applied to a strong benevolent, the sick is easily recovered; for the weakest always goes to the wall.

11. If Saturn be signifier of the sickness, oriental of the Sun, the disease coming of cold, etc., occidental of the Sun, the disease coming of heat, seldom kills: My Author may be something questioned for this; yet this I'll easily grant him, that Saturn is not so subject to take away life in such a life as in the contrary. I dare not be positive in the thing, because I have not spoken with Dr. Experience about it.

12. Mars is not so formidable when he is occidental as when he is oriental.

13. Mars afflicts the Moon more when she is oriental than he does when she is occidental.

14. A reception between the Lord of the Ascendent and the Lord of the eighth, if they be benevolent, or if the benevolence lend them aid, shows recovery.

15. Also my Author says that if the Lord of the eighth receives the Lord of the Ascendent without the malicious beams of ill fortunes, the sick will escape, even when there is no hope of life.

16. I know not the truth of it, because as yet I know not the judgment of Dr. Experience in the thing; but Dr. Reason is of opinion that it is far better that the Lord of the Ascendent dispose the Lord of the eighth than that the Lord of the eighth dispose the Lord of the Ascendent.

17. Is it not better that life dispose of death than that death dispose of life? Indeed this he told me, that if the Lord of the Ascendent does dispose the Lord of the eighth, the sick will take such a course as will be for his own prejudice, and the hastening on of his end.

18. But if sick people will not be ruled by fair means, they must be ruled by foul; and that is all that I can say unto it.

19. If good Planets be in the Ascendent or Mid-heaven at the decumbiture, and pretty strong withall, they will stand to their tackling stoutly to maintain life, though the signifiers of it be never so much afflicted.

Part 3: Signs of Death.

1. First of all, the Lord of the Ascendent afflicted in the eighth, the Patient is more mad to be *apud inferos,* than death is to have him; the man will die, and his life will be cast away absolutely with evil guidance.

2. If at the Decumbiture you find the Lord of the ascendent, combust in the ascendent, pass the same judgment with the former.

3. If the Lord of the eighth house be in the mid-heavens, and afflict the Lord of the Ascendent, the Physic will be in a shrewd mistake, and instead of curing go near to kill.

4. Listen to this, O College of Physicians; let me entreat you to learn the principles of your trade; and I beseech you no longer mistake avarice for wit and honesty.

5. The Lord of the eighth, very strong in the Ascendent, gives you fair warning that death's a coming.

6. A conjunction between the Lord of the eighth and the Lord of the Ascendent is as mortal a sign as the Lord of the heavens can show.

7. It is a very unlucky sign when the Lord of the eighth house is Lord of the house at the decumbiture. And not much better if the Lord of

the house at the decumbiture be afflicted by the Lord of the eighth; especially if the Lord of the eighth be a malevolent.

8. Such ill beginning of a disease usually proves fatal at the latter end, unless the Physician be a very able man.

9. If the Lord of the Ascendent fall retrograde from the body of the Lord of the eighth, it gives you a timely warning of death at their next conjunction, unless the Lord of the ascendent meet with the

10. Sun before he meet with the Lord of death again.

11. The Lord of the eighth in conjunction square, or opposition to the Moon at the decumbiture, threatens death, unless there be a reception between them. If the Lord of the eight be retrograde or infortunated, you may the more confide in his judgment.

12. The Lord of the eighth in an angle, especially the western angle, the Moon and Lord of the ascendent being in cadent houses or afflicted by malevolents; death may be feared, and that justly too; especially if a malevolent be in the eighth, or Lord of that house.

13. The Moon, with both Saturn and Jupiter, profits not the sick at all, unless Jupiter be much stronger than Saturn, or with the Lord of the Ascendent than either of them.

14. In such a case medicines under the influence of Jupiter will do good, because his body is afflicted by so potent an adversary.

15. This had I from Dr. Reason; neither is it barely to assist him of truth, but a foundation to build other truths upon; a rule for practice; a key to open the closet of practice; a heurete to find other truths by.

16. The Lord of the ascendent in the aspect, or with the antiscion of an infortune in the eighth, threatens death, unless the wholesome beams of Jupiter and Venus help; which if, there will be a strong contest between nature and the disease.

17. The fortunes strive to maintain nature, the infortunes to destroy them: in such a case, look which is strongest, and pass judgment upon the end of the dispute accordingly.

18. If you find the Moon in like case in an acute disease, or the Sun in a Chronical, pass the same judgment.

19. If there be a reception between the Lord of the ascendent, and the Lord of the eighth by any aspect, the sick will probably live; and that as I remember I told you before. But the sickness will be long and tedious, and the effects of it lie long in the body, and that I never told you till now.

20. The Moon with Saturn and Mars, or the Moon with the one, and the Sun with the other, or either of them with one, and the Lord of the ascendent with the other, or the Lord of the ascendent with both, gives shrewd suspicions, that the sickness is but the Prodomus or usherer in of death.

21. The slower in motion the afflicting infortune is, the worse it is; for then the Moon meets him again upon the Critical day.

22. The Lord of the ascendent in the seventh or fourth houses, and there afflicted, gives warning to the sick man that his dissolution is at hand.

23. An infortune upon the Cusp of the Horoscope bids the sick provide for a change.

24. Fixed stars of a violent nature, speak the same language, if they be upon the Horoscope.

25. Those fixed stars are said to be of a violent nature, which are of the nature of Saturn or Mars; as Lanx

Australis, the Bull's eyes, the Scorpion's heart, etc., and some which are of the nature of the fortunes, if Authors mistake not their natures, as Algol, or the head of Medusa, which is placed in the Buckler of Perseus. The Grecian Astrologers call him the Devil's-head; and yet all the Astrologers, Jupiter and Venus to have a share in his nature. Let it suffice that all hold, and Doctor Experience himself certifies, that his conditions are as bad as who is worst. Neither shall he come behind any one of the fixed stars in doing mischief.

26. If the Moon be void of course at the beginning of the sickness, and yet afflicted upon a critical day, a good Crisis cannot be hoped; an ill Crisis may justly be feared and that not without grounds from sober rules of Art.

27. The Lord of the ascendent in Leo or Aquarius impedited by the body of the Lord of the 6th or 12th houses, signifies danger of death.

28. Both the Luminaries afflicted under the earth carry the same signification.

29. It is evil if the Moon be in a detriment or fall at the Crisis, though she be not afflicted at all; the time of the Crisis is the time of a combat between nature and the disease.

30. And if the Moon be weak, she is not able to maintain nature in the combat.

31. The Sun afflicted by the body Square or Opposition or Antiscion of a malevolent, it tells the patient the disease will be long and tedious, if not mortal; and bids him provide himself of such a Physician as knows how to do something else besides only to tell money.

32. The Moon opposed to the Lord of the ascendent at the beginning of a sickness, if the Lord of the

ascendent be also retrograde or combust, shows bitter accidents will fall out to the sick during the time of his sickness;

33. He is a wise Physician that can remedy them; but he is wise that can anticipate them.

34. The Moon in the fourth house with the body square, opposition or antiscion of Mars, soon brings a man to his last inheritance, the Grave; she threatens it, if she be there no way afflicted, unless he be very strong.

35. As I have judged by the Moon, so judge by Mars if you find him; for if he being there have any dignities in the ascendent, he will urge a man as fast to his grave as ever sleep urged him to bed.

36. Saturn opposite to the Lord of the eighth house threatens danger enough to the sick.

37. The Moon in Conjunction with Mars in the fourth house will send the sick to take a supper in another world, though both their fortunes stand and look upon him.

38. The Moon in the ascendent, if you will believe Authors, always hurts; and they give some show of reason of it, because there she has most power over the body of the sick.

39. Yet mine own opinion for the present is, that if she be there, and in Cancer or Taurus, she will rather help than hinder the sick. If the Moon does hate the ascendent as Authors say, I suppose the reason to be because Saturn loves it. And then she hates the eighth and twelfth houses by the same rule. And if you will call your wits into examination, they will tell you it is true enough.

40. If the Moon be in the ascendent, and the sign ascending of a contrary nature to her, it is a hundred to one that the sick die not of that disease.

41. And here my Author spoke something to the purpose: If the former Aphorism made a discord in your brain, this, if rightly understood, will reduce them to a harmony.

42. The Moon applying to the body of the Sun, within twelve degrees at the Decumbiture, the sickness comes not so much to terrify your body, as to give you warning of your end.

43. And the nearer the Moon is to the body of the Sun, the speedier dispatch will death make of the body of his captive.

44. The Moon besieged by the bodies of the malevolents positive between the Sun and one of them, the hopes of life are very small, or none at all.

45. Authors say that if a man or woman fall sick when the Moon is going out of combustion, their sickness will increase till she comes to the opposition of the Sun. And if then she meet with an ill Planet, the sick recovers; if not, they die. For mine own particular, I speak no more than I have found by continual experience; I have often found this false and never true.

46. If the Sun or Moon be Lord of the house at the decumbiture, and behold the Lord of the eighth; the sickness is sent to proclaim the approach of death.

47. It is very bad when the Moon carries the light of the lord of the ascendent to the lord of the eighth, it threatens death; but it does not so in all diseases neither; for example, in such as come and go by fits, as Agues, falling sickness, etc., you may make this use of it; that none are fit to make Physicians, but such as are intimately acquainted with Madam Nature, and her eldest son Dr. Reason.

48. It is extremely bad when the Moon applies to any star in the eighth, as bad as when she applies to the lord of the eighth himself.

49. The Moon combust in the eighth in Leo, threatens death, says my Author; and so the truth is she does, if she be combust in any other house or sign, unless she separate from the body of the Sun.

50. The disease will appear little otherwise than the forerunner of death, if the Moon be in Libra, and Jupiter and Venus in conjunction; he that knows anything in Physic that he should know, knows the reason well enough.

51. The Moon with the Pleiades, and the Aries, or with any other violent fixed star, shows danger of death.

52. The Moon applying to her own Nodes, namely the head and tail of the Dragon is very bad, but not so bad if she separates from them.

53. It is very bad when Saturn is in his Apogeon, or near it, if the disease come of retention.

54. Judge the like by Mars, if the disease be a fever, or proceed of choler; and here you have another instructor to teach you knowledge; the nearer a planet is to the earth, the more stoutly will he maintain and increase the humors he governs.

55. It is a very bad sign, if not disparate, if there be an Eclipse of either Luminary upon a critical day; and if it miss a day of it, it will break no squares in such a case: the time of the Eclipse has to my

56. knowledge anticipated the time of the Crisis a whole day natural, and proved mortal too, as I have had experience in Essex, in the latter end of October, 1649.

57. Thus have I given you the signs of death, by Astrology; I do not say absolutely a man must needs

die when any of these signs appear; but this I say, the danger of death is much; I advise the Physician to have a care what he does; let him advise with nature, and her two sons, Doctor Reason and Doctor Experience; let him have some brains in his head and not all in his books; let the Patient provide for a change, and make his peace with God, and set his house in order, and then has he the less need to care whether he live or die.

One Chapter of Noel Duryet, which is the last, and contains certain observations taken out of Cardanus and other expert Physicians, which at first I intended to translate, but finding them very imperfect, I thought good to forbear, for wanting an Ephemerides of that age to perfect them myself, I thought better to leave them quite out than trouble this prying age with imperfections.

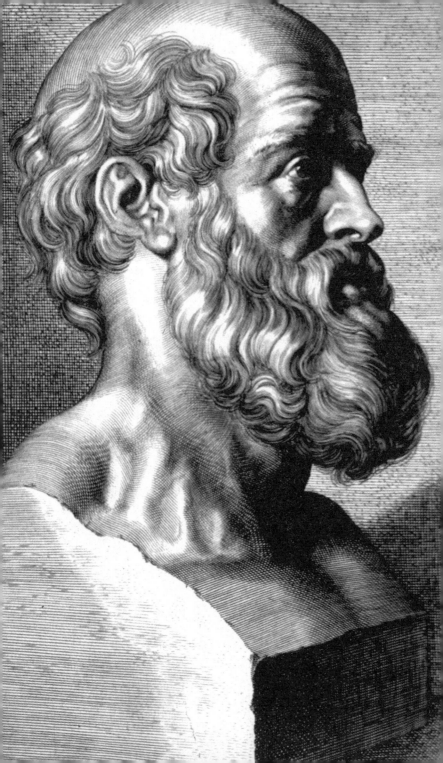

Hippocrates' Presages of life and death, by the body of the patient being sick.

T wo ways did the famous Hippocrates leave to posterity for the judging of the life and death of sick people: one by the celestial aspects of the Planets, and the other by the Symptoms of the body of the man lying sick. The latter of these must first be performed; the profit of which, for 'tis good for something, according to Hippocrates, is first the credit of the Physician: so first of all, he hence avoid defamation, evil speeches and reproaches; the world shall never say he is a Dunce.

It will better his own knowledge, he need not apply living medicines to a dying man. Secondly, for the profit of the sick; hereby you may give them warning of death before it comes, and they will the more confidently commit themselves to the hands of a Physician when they know he knows something.

If the credit of Hippocrates may pass for starling, he protests that what I here write, was confirmed in all his practices in Ethiopia, Libya, Mauritania, the Isle of Delos, Scythia, and Italy.

And he that diligently observes these, and compares them with the aspects of heavenly bodies, can never without a miracle fail in his judgment upon diseases. For my own part, I dare command the greatest part of them for authentic, though I have not made trial of them all; yet 'tis very probable, set the antiquity of the Author aside, that the meanest of them (if well heeded) may give a more infallible judgment upon a disease than a whole Tub-full of Physicians.

I have somewhat inverted Hippocrates' order; and my reason was because I would bring the business into one single ingress, and make them as plain to the meanest capacity as a pikestaff: and if they cannot understand them, as I have committed them to posterity, the fault is in the dullness of their own wits, and there let it rest.

Hippocrates divides them into three books, and in that I will follow him to a hair.

The first book I shall divide into these parts: presages of diseases.

1. The face.
2. The eyes and lips.
3. The manner of lying.
4. The teeth.
5. Ulcers or Issues.
6. The Hands.
7. The breath.
8. The sweat.
9. Tumors and Apostumes.

Presages by the Face.

If in a sick body the face look as it did in the time of health, or but little different; the hope of recovery is not small: signs of death in the face of a sick body, are these:

1. The Nostrils are extenuated and very sharp.
2. The Eyes are hollow.
3. The skin of the forehead or eyebrows, hard, dry, and loose; and looks as though it were tan'd.
4. The Ears are cold, shrunk, and almost doubled.
5. The face is black, pale, or swarthy, or deformed; he looks but ill-favoredly.

If these, or most of these, appear (be not to rash neither for rashness is the daughter of ignorance; but be sober minded; and first inquire whether the Patient have not fasted much, or wanted sleep, or had a flux a long time: if these, or any of these, had not a being before the sickness, the danger of death is to be feared.

If the sickness has been four or five days before you see these Symptoms, they are but the harbingers of death, and he follows them at the tail.

Presages by the Eyes and Lips.

1. Signs of death by the eyes are, if they be deprived of sight, or weep against the patient's will.

2. If they seem as though they would fall out of his head.

3. When one of the eyes becomes less than the other.

4. When the white of the eyes become reddish.

5. When they are bleary-eyed, or dim-eyed, and not used to be so before.

6. When they are very moveable, gashful, staring up and down, or sunk deep into the head.

7. When the sick grows squint eyed, and not so before, and stares up and down as though he was frightened.

8. When the Patient sleeps with his eyes open, and was not so accustomed to do.

9. Then inquire if these come not by flux, nor laxative medicines; if not, they are signs of death.

10. When the Eyelids, Nose, and Lips are crooked, or drawn in to one side.

11. If the lips are thin, cold, pale, and hanging down, and the nose very sharp, it denotes death.

Presages by the manner of lying in Bed.

It is best when men lie in bed in that form in sickness as they did when they were in health, mortal signs are first.

1. When the neck, hands, and feet are extended, stiff and inflexible, not to be moved.

2. Sudden starting up out of the bed.

3. Casting their head down to the feet of the bed.

4. Sleeping with their mouth open contrary to former custom.

5. Tossing and tumbling, or throwing himself from one end of the bed to the other, shows the man in a terrible condition, if not in a dying condition.

6. To sleep with the belly downward, contrary to custom, shows aches of the belly, or little less than madness.

7. If the desire in sickness be to go out of one room into another, mistake the room for a world.

8. He that is impatient and forces himself to rise upon a Critical day puts himself in great danger: if the disease be violent and touch his Lungs, the Critical day may prove mortal.

Presages by the teeth.

1. Gnashing of the teeth in a Fever, if not naturally, is a dangerous sign.

2. If with all he be deprived of his senses, and his sickness, only a Fever not a frenzy, and gnashes his teeth, he calls for death, and he will quickly come.

Presages by Ulcers and Issues.

If a sick person has any Ulcer or issue, whether it came before the sickness or with it; (there is not a half penny to choose) and it will dry up and become green, black, or swarthy if the Patient becomes worse and worse, Doctor Death is coming to cure him.

Presages by the Hands.

If in Fevers or any other acute diseases, frenzy excepted, the sick by pedaling or plucking the bed-clothes, or pulling straws if he could find them, a thousand to one if he lives the age of a little fish. Judge the like, if he takes violent hold of the bed-clothes, ceiling, or wall.

Presages by the Breath.

By the breath is best judgment given upon the spirits, heart, and lungs.

If a disease has invaded the spirits (and that is the quickest way to kill a man), carry a urinal full of Piss to the Doctor, and he will say he ails nothing; the reason is, there is no digestion found in the urine; because the disease seizes not the body, but the spirits. A man is troubled in mind, his Wife and Children do not please him; being troubled, is sick for madness; his wife, as bad as she is, loves him, and as ill as she hates him, she will carry his Piss to the Doctor; he looks upon it, and thinks the man is as well as himself (and that is bad enough), only his trouble is not so great: he knows as much by his urine, as if he had looked into a Crow's nest; he has no more skill in Astrology than I have in making of Candles; the man speaks out all his wit at once, and [the wife] says her husband ails nothing; it may be 'tis true enough, he ails nothing, but only to be out of this world; the drift of this discourse is only to show you some diseases seize only upon the spirits, others only upon the body. But to the purpose.

The distance between breathing, if it be too long, and coldness of the breath, shows death is not above two or three feet off; gentle breath in hot diseases, is an argument of death.

Presages by Sweat.

1. Those kind sweats which happen upon judicial or critical days, are wholesome, commendable, and good, for they are sent by Doctor Health.

2. If sweat be universal, 'tis excellent; and if the Patient mends by his sweating, 'tis a forerunner of a Cure.

3. Mortal sweats are first of all cold.

4. Only in one part of the body, usually in the forehead and face; if the Patient afflicted by such sweats dies not, his diseases will continue longer than he would have it.

Presages by tumors.

1. If the Patient that lies sick of a Fever, feels neither pain, inflammation, tumor, nor hardness upon or near about his Ribs, 'tis a very good sign.

2. If any of these be there, and upon both sides, 'tis but a bad sign at the best.

3. If he feels great motions and pulsations in one of his sides, it prognosticates great pain and deprivation of his senses.

4. If with his pulsation his eyes move faster than they should do, the Patient is in danger to fall into a frenzy, if not to mischief himself.

The last Chapter of Apostumes.

1. The Collection of an Apostume in both sides in a burning Fever, is more dangerous than if it had been but upon one side; for two men will sooner kill a man than one.

2. 'Tis more dangerous on the left side than on the right.

3. If it continues 20 days, and the Fever ceases not, neither the Apostumes deminish, it will come to mature action.

4. If there comes a Flux of blood through the nose upon the first critical day, it eases the Patient; only he will be pained in his head, and troubled with dimness of sight at noon day, chiefly if he be about thirty, or thirty five, years of age.

5. When the Apostume is soft, and with pain when 'tis handled, it requires a longer time to cure than the former did, but not half so dangerous.

6. Such a one may continue two months before it comes to be ripe.

7. That Apostume that is hard, great, and painful, if it be not mortal, I am sure it is dangerous.

8. Apostumes of the belly are never so great as those that grow under the midriff; and yet those that grow under the Navel are less than they, and usually come to suppuration.

9. 'Tis a good sign when they purge by a Flux of blood in the nostrils.

10. Some Apostumes purge only outwards, and they are little round and sharp pointed; and they are most healthful, less mortal.

11. Such as are large, gross, not round but flat, are most dangerous.

12. Those that purge and break within the belly, and make tumors outwardly, are as bad as the Devil himself, or Robin Good-fellow, and are very pernicious, those that make no tumor outwardly, excel them as far as the shot of a Cannon does that of a Pistol.

13. The matter which comes out of the impostumes, being white and not unsavory, is very good and healthful.

14. The more the color differs from white, the worse it is; and thus much for the first book.

The second Book of the Presages of Hippocrates, you shall find marshaled in this Order:

Presages by dropsies in Fevers

1. First, all manner of Dropsies in Fevers are dangerous, if not mortal: I know you would fain

know a reason; I'll tell you: a Fever proceeds of heat, Dropsies of cold; and as fire and water agree, so does a Fever and a Dropsy; and what you give to mitigate a Fever, increases a Dropsy; a Dropsy and a Fever agree like fire and water; the Sun having drawn up a fiery quality from the earth, and enveloped it round with a cloud of Snow; thence comes lightning and thunder, and terrifies the people; and as well does a Fever and a Dropsy agree in Microcosms, as fire and water does in the Region of the air; many men know their is a middle Region in the air, but few know what it is, and as little where, only a few Sons whom mother Wisdom has instructed in it.

2. If a Dropsy and a Fever meet in one body, they will play wreaks (as sometimes they do, though not often), the Liver pays all the score.

3. It afflicts the *Vena lectua*, and most commonly the guts themselves; the legs are presently tormented, and they cannot march handsomely; a flux follows, and the swelling in the belly is not a whit lessened by it.

4. If the Liver be most afflicted, the Patient has got a dry cough, and he knows not how to help it; he spits but very little, and wishes he could spit more; the belly is very hard, and if he goes to stool, 'tis with more pain than he would willing; his feet swell, there are tumors, inflammation in his sides; sometimes they dissipate, and sometimes they swell again.

Presages of Life and Death in Fevers.

1. When the Patient is cold on his head or face, or has cold sweats there; also if his hands and feet be cold, but his belly and sides hot and burning, the case is extreme dangerous, and is a sign that death

has taken possession of the house and clay where life formerly dwelt.

2. It is a healthful sign in a Fever, when all the parts of the body are equally hot, though they be something hotter than they should be.

3. The body heavy, the nails of a leaden swarthy color, the disease will be cured by death, and not by Physic.

4. Enduring a sickness without anguish, shows strength of nature; and so long as she hold up her head, there is some hope.

5. Let every one that views a Patient, if he would act the part of a wise man, inquire after the custom of the man's body when he was in health; and if his spittle, sleep, or excrement etc. be as they were when the body was in health, recovery is coming, and it comes a pace, and will speedily be with the sick for his comfort.

6. The more these signs differ in sickness from what they were in health, the more is the danger.

7. By these signs you may also know in some measure what part of the body is afflicted, and by what humor if you can but understand their language; if you cannot, go to the school of dame Nature, she is an excellent School-Mistress.

Presages by the Testicles.

When the yard and testicles are shrunk in, and apparently diminished against nature, it signifies great pain and anguish, and death follows them at heels as swift as the wind.

Presages of Sleeping.

1. First of all, when the sick sleeps in the night, and keeps waking in the day, this is usually a lovely hopeful sign of recovery to the sick; the reins of

government are not yet forced out of the hands of dame Nature; and if she be not hindered by intemperance or other impediments, governs prudently.

2. Although it be not altogether wholesome to sleep from break of day till eight or nine of the clock in the morning; yet it is more commendable to sleep than than any other time of the day.

3. Continual watching is extremely dangerous, and cries aloud that deprivation of senses is at hand, if it be not already come.

Presages by the Excrements of the Belly in fevers.

1. First of all, the most commendable sign is when he that is surprised with a fever retains the same custom in avoiding his excrements, which he ordinarily used when his body was best in health.

2. Always in excrements you must regard the quality and quantity of the diet; for take this for a certain rule, and you shall find it never varies without a miracle, how much the excrements are different from that, so much worse is the sign.

3. Laudable excrements are neither too thick nor too thin, yet it is worse that they be too thick than too thin; for astringency in a fever is naught and not to be allowed. He is fitter to make a Hangman than a Physician that takes no care that his Patient go orderly to stool.

4. A looseness in a fever proclaims to the world that the Patient kept ill diet before.

5. It is exceedingly good that the color of the excrements be according to the food taken.

6. It is very good that the patient go to stool without pain; for if nature be troubled to expel natural excrements, she will find a harder pull of it to expel the disease.

7. If the excrements be liquid, viz. if the man that is sick of a fever has a looseness, and what comes from him, comes without violence, pain or wind, it is a hopeful sign, for nature has found out a way to turn out the disease at the back-door.

8. Yet I beseech you, take notice of this; frequent going to stool weakens the sick, spoils the digestion, mars the retentive faculty, makes the sick froward and faint.

9. Worms coming forth of the body with excrements, at the end of the Malady is a good sign and hopeful. But at the beginning of the sickness 'tis desperate; the poor worms know when nature is a decaying, and therefore leave the body before it is breathless.

10. Here's a strange thing, that the worms have as much knowledge as the Physician.

11. It's very good in every sickness, when the belly is soft, and not puffed up with wind; wind is an active creature, and plays wreaks in the body of man when it gets where it should not be.

12. The excrements when they are very watery, white, or very red or frothy they are very dangerous.

13. But by the leave of Hippocrates, not always mortal.

14. Excrements black, green, or slimy give you fair warning, if any warning will serve the turn, that the disease may end in death, and that's most probable.

15. Mixture of the forenamed colors is no less dangerous, but shows longer continuance of the disease, in the former the sick runs to his grave as

hard as he can drive; in this he walks to the same place as though he told his steps.

16. When little skins like the peeling of guts come forth of the excrements, the disease is dangerous. This symptom was ordinarily seen, in that Epidemical disease in London 1649 which so puzzled the College of Physicians, that their learned ignorance was so far from curing of it, that they could not tell what it was.

17. Then Master Galen (for they know not where dame nature the Mother of Physicians dwells) instructed them in no such principles.

18. Mine own Son, about three years of age, was taken of the same disease, myself in the Country; when the hopes of life were but small, I was sent for up; what came from him, and that was once in an hour, was wrapped round in skins.

19. I cured him by only boiling Mallows in his drink; and to manifest my thankfulness to God, for so great a mercy, I here declare it to the world.

Presages by wind in the Bowels and Womb.

1. First of all, wind issuing forth gently and voluntarily, is the best and most wholesome sign.

2. Worse than that when it comes forth with pain and griping.

3. Worst of all when it is retained, and cannot come out at all, but causes swellings there.

4. Swellings of the wind in the belly according to Hippocrates, are best cured by expulsion downward, or by Urine; thus my Author.

I care not greatly if I relate the cure done in such a case by one of the wisest Physicians that ever the Sun shone upon in

England, Dr. Butler of Cambridge. A Gentleman was possessed with wind in his belly, a great inflammation there was there. The Doctor comes to him, and perceiving the original of it was wind; for he was a man of penetrating judgment, calling for a rolling pin. The man was never subject to covetousness, and as little to pride: down turns he the clothes from the bed: up he gets boots and all, not regarding the holland sheets; and falls to rolling the man's belly with a Rolling-pin; the Patient's fundament sounds an alarm, and certifies all the company that ease was a coming.

Presages by the Urine in fevers.

1. First of all, if the Urine in a fever or any other sickness has residence near the bottom, in color white, in form like a Pyramid.

2. So much the more the Urine differs from this, so much the worse it is.

3. Gross resolutions, like dust or bran in the bottom of the Urine, is a very evil sign.

4. But 'tis worse than that, when they are like scales of fish.

5. The Urine white and clear, signifies melancholy, and is very bad; for if the retentive faculty be caused by melancholy, the disease is like enough to hold long; for melancholy will retain as well what it should not as what it should.

6. A cloud hanging in the Urine signifies health if it be white; if it be black 'tis dangerous; and then your Mother wit will tell you that the blacker it is, it is the more dangerous.

7. The Urine yellow very clear and subtle, shows the sickness will continue longer than the sick party would willingly have it; crudity and indigestion has taken occasion to shoulder out health.

8. In such a case there is fear, and that not a little, least the sick die before the humor come to concoction; what a trick's that to cut off nature before she can do her business? And let me tell you this, I knew a man in London that shall be nameless, that was surprised with a furious and merciless pestilential fever; his Urine was according to this Aphorism, he had a swelling in his Emunctuary of the brain, (viz.) under his hair.

9. It rose as fairly as fair could be, even till the hour of his death, yet he died; nature did the best she could to expel the disease, but she was anticipated; did you never know a man die in the prime of his health? If not, go to St. Tyburne and you may be informed.

10. Slimy, muddy, black, tawny, dirty, nasty, filthy, stinking urine is usually mortal.

11. If a child's urine be brought to you, and it looks pale and clear, like conduit water, it is very bad; I know you long for a reason, you shall not lose your longing; I told you before such a humor was the badge of a melancholy disposition; youth is naturally hot and moist; melancholy cold and dry; ergo, extreme inimical to youth.

12. If you spy in the Urine a thing like a cob-web swimming on the top, it is but a scurvy sign.

13. Thick Urine signifies but a thin body, for he that made it has a consumption.

14. White clouds in the urine and near the bottom are commendable; black clouds and near the top are bad and vituperous.

In all these have regard to the bladder; for if that be diseased, all these presages are in vain.

Thus Hippocrates; the truth is, many of them seem to me pretty rational; neither am I able to contradict the rest, as I have never been a piss-Prophet all my life; yet this I know to be true, and Dr. Experience is my witness, that if the man be sick of a fever, and the urine appears like the urine of a healthy man, as I have known it in more than one, and by this argument will I prove a very uncertainty in urine, death's coming, provide for him.

I spake with Dr. Reason at the same time for they two brethren seldom go asunder, and he told me the reason was because the disease worked upon the spirits, and not upon the body: and that's as ready a way to kill a man as to chop off his head.

Presages of Vomiting in fevers.

1. First to vomit up phlegm and choler in a fever is a very good sign, because they are better out of your body than in it; they are but scurvy inmates when they keep not their proper place.

2. If what is vomited up be green, livid, or black, 'tis dangerous.

3. If it be mixed or compounded of these, 'tis mortal.

4. If it stinks, so that you cannot endure to hold your nose over it, and have but one of these colors, death comes galloping; thus Hippocrates.

Hippocrates was a brave Physician, I confess; Galen mended his works in Physic, just as Aristotle mended Plato's in Philosophy, and that is as sour Ale mends in Summer.

Presages by the Spittle in fevers.

1. Spittle in all diseases of the lungs, and maladies under the ribs, if it come in the beginning of the disease, without pain, of such a color as spittle should be, well digested, not viscous, It's very commendable, there's some hopes of it.

2. If the spittle come not up without vehement coughing; it's an ill sign when nature is forced by violence to cast out her enemy.

3. White spittle, tough and knotty, is very dangerous in a fever; but when men spit blood, it's worse, and yet such things happen sometimes.

4. If the Spittle be green or fleshy, it gives notice of a bad and ill conditioned sickness.

5. Black spittle is the worst of all, for then grim death's a coming.

6. When the matter which should be spit out, remains still within the lungs and troubles the windpipe, there's but little security of life: and I am confident never a one of the college keeps an insurance office for such a business, nor will insure thereupon at 50 percent.

7. What we told you was wholesome at the beginning of the malady, if it continue longer than the first Crisis, it's suspicious, if it be not dangerous.

8. If the pain be eased by spitting, it's very good; let the wind blow which way it will; and then

9. If the Spittle be black, and if spittle does foreshadow death, it is that yet if the pain be eased by it, though I cannot say it is hopeful, yet this I say, it is less dangerous.

Presages by Sneezing in fevers.

1. Sneezing in hot maladies (let the malady be as dangerous as a halter); it is hopeful and commendable, and may procure a Reprieve.

2. Yet in maladies of the lungs, if it come with much rheum, and pain be felt after, it is dangerous, come it when it will, whether in the fit or presently after.

Presages of Suppuration of Apostumes.

1. If the pain of an Apostume cease not by spitting, to which add laxative medicines, and letting blood, 'tis forty to one if it come not to suppuration.

2. When the Apostume breaks, the spittle, giving notice of choler, whether matter come out with the spittle, or after, it is dangerous.

3. If the matter come upon the first Crisis, it comes to tell you death will come upon the second Crisis, unless the Physician be all the wiser to stave him off: does there such a one live in Amen-Corner?

4. If the former Aphorism appear, and other healthful signs appear together with it, Dame Nature may happen to help herself, and never be beholding to the College: and if you be ruled by me, take acquaintance with her; and that you may do so, I'll describe her to you, that you may know her when you meet her in the street: she's a plain, homely woman in a beggarly contemptible condition, regarded by none (unless it be the children of wisdom); she has truth written upon her breast; those that think themselves wise tread her underfoot; she carries Dr. Reason in her right hand, and Dr. Experience in her left; her head is bound about with the eternal providence, and in her brain is written the knowledge of all things, in words at length and not in figures: she always goes toward heaven; and if you ask her, she'll bid you come after: God is her Father, and her Mother's name is the good of the Creation. If you follow her you shall not want: she treads upon the world, and looks upwards: she is a virgin, a wife, and a widow: she will give you a paper in your hand, in which is written, Know thyself: she has no money, yet is Mistress of the mines of India. In all her words you shall find more truth than eloquence:

If you please to ask her for her Commission, she will show it you, signed by Jebovah, not by Aristotle or Galen. Her ways are very plain, you may find them in the darkest night without a Candle and lantern; she is always everywhere and yet still with me: she is my Mother; she's a woman and yet an Academic: she's present to all that call upon her, yet not Ubiquitary: she always weeps, and yet I never saw her laugh. I hope none will blame me for writing this description of my Mother, so much despised, so little thought of by the Rabbis of our age. *Noverint universi per praesentes*, that she is my Mother; and her two Sons, Dr. Reason, and Dr. Experience, my brethren.

Presages by the time of the Ruptures of Apostumes.

1. That all Apostumes have not one and the same time of maturation, is so certain that it needs no further dispute of the story.

2. It is most usual and most wholesome for Apostumes to break upon judicial days; what they be and when they happen you know already, unless you began at the latter end of the Book first. Hippocrates reckons them by number of days, 'tis true; but so have not I, but by the course of the Moon. Do not blame Hippocrates for a small fault; rather think yourselves engaged to him for doing anything; it may be 'twas Galen's fault, not his.

3. Take notice that Hippocrates was guided by good principles; for he tells you, that the beginning of the disease is when the Patient feels heat, a fever, stiffness, pain, pricking, or anything else that denotes a disease.

4. When you feel that, do but so much for me as to make that time the basis to prognosticate the event.

5. Coughing, spitting, and spawling, pain, difficulty of breathing, are true prognostics that the Apostume is near breaking.

6. As by the Forlorn-hope you may judge what the Army is; so by these signs you may judge of the greatness of the Apostume.

7. As by a Citizen's spending you may judge how long he will hold; so by the swiftness of these signs you may judge how soon the Apostume will break.

8. Sometimes the Apostume breaks, and life is undone by it; sometimes it breaks, and death runs away for fear of the noise. 'Twere worth the while to know how this might be known. I'll tell you how, and never go so far as an Amen-Corner for it neither.

9. If when the Apostumes break the man begins to fall to his victuals, and feed like a Farmer; if the matter be white, equal, salt, and come out without pain; take these to be signs of speedy health, and say I told you so.

10. If the fever cease not, or ceasing come with a fresh supply, 'twere worth the while to know whether it will return again or no, I'll tell you how to know (if you will but read it). If the fever will return again, the thirst remains still to keep possession: and when the fever does return again, the Feces being very watery, green, livid or slimy, fortify against death; for he is not far off.

11. If the Patient feel pain on both sides, both sides are Apostumated; wherefore do they ask else think you?

12. If he feel more pain on one side than on the other, cause him to lie on the soundest side. If he feel heaviness there, be sure there is an Apostume also.

13. If some good signs appear, and some bad, compare them all together, and judge by most testimony;

make use of all the rules you can, that so you may find the truth, and avoid infamy.

Presages of Apostumes about the Ears.

1. First, when Apostumes which come either about or under the ears come to maturation and break, the bitterness of death is past.

2. You may know when there's an Aposthume there by swelling and pain, by heat and burning, by redness of color and inflammation about the place.

Apostumes in the feet.

1. In vehement and dangerous diseases of the lungs, it conduces much to the help of the Patient when small pustules or Apostumes appear in the feet.

2. If withall the spittle change from red to white, it gives certain testimony that recovery approaches.

3. If the spittle turns not from red to white, then the pain ceases not, and the sinews of the part apostumated, are in danger of shrinking.

4. If together with the former, the Apostumes also vanish away, the man loses his senses first, and his life afterwards.

5. Aged people are more usually troubled with the diseases in the lungs than young people.

6. It's very dangerous in all Apostumes, when the pain ascends upwards.

7. Easy spitting white spittle, and not stinking, is a commendable sign in all diseases of the lungs; but if your spittle be red, black, or stinking, 'tis deadly.

Presages by the Bladder in Fevers.

1. First, hardness and pain in the Bladder in quotidian Fevers, usually foreshadows death is approaching.

2. If withal the urine be stopped, judge the like.

3. In Apostumes of the Bladder (when they come in scurvy places), if the urine be like matter of the Apostume, and the pain cease, and the Fever mitigate, and the Bladder be mollified; when you see these signs, you may be confident the worst is past.

4. This disease usually happens to few, but Children, and to them most usually, about the 7th or 14th year of their age.

The third Book of the Presages of Hippocrates.

This book I confess is but short, yet the better order it is in, the handsomer will I look; and the reason is, because God is the God of Order.

Let no man blame that Gallant soul Hippocrates for writing a little disorderly; rather let him bless God that he wrote at all: Let our College of Physicians write so to purpose, and in their Mother tongue as he did in his; and the rest of my days shall be spent in admiring and applauding of them.

But to return to my purpose, you shall find this third book presented to your view in this Order.

1. Presages in Fevers.

2. Quinsies.

3. The Uvula.

4. Vomiting in Fevers.

Of all these in Order.

Presages in Fevers.

1. This is most certain, and verified by continual experience, that a Fever terminates in death to one, and in life to another, in both upon one and the same days and the reason why, you may find in the beginning of this book in that part, the basest of which was borrowed from the famous Avenezra.

2. Then you see a reason why it is as requisite to view the body of the sick, as the position of the stars.

   It is a custom in Italy, or at least it was but a few years since, that a Physician might not deny to view a sick body, if he had but his fee given him, which amounted but to 18 d. ster; if he carry two Scholars with him, he had 12. d. more, if the Patient were willing to give it him; which being added to the former, amounts just to 3 s. 6 d. if he carried twenty Scholars, he had no more.

3. To the Patient comes he, for he dare not deny it what ere the disease be; if he be in health, and at liberty, there does he instruct the Scholars by the Urine, by the Symptoms of the disease, it's continuation and accidents etc. whether the sick be like to live or die, how the disease opposes nature, and which way.

4. This makes the Italian Physicians able men, when the greatest part of ours are like to die dunces; who dares deny, that has but wit to know his right hand from his left, but that seeing the body, hearing the relation, and feeling the pulse of the sick, is a better way to judge than gazing upon as much piss as the Thames will hold?

5. I wish from my heart our present State would take this matter into consideration, and take a little care for the lives of the poor Commonalty, that a poor man that wants money to buy his wife and Children

bread, may not perish for want of an angel to fee a proud insulting domineering Physician, to give him a Visit. I think it is a duty belonging to the Keepers of the Liberty of England. I would help my poor brethren in this particular if I could, but I cannot.

6. Whosoever reads what I have here written, and approves of it; let him join with me in a Petition to the State, for the rectifying of this disorder.

7. Those which approve not of it, let them answer me to this question: who made a difference between the Rich and the poor? Was it God or the world?

8. If the world, as is most certain, then will it not stand; for the fashion of the world passes away.

9. If many good signs appear at the beginning of a Fever, note the sign and degree the moon is in at the Decumbiture. And the party will recover when the moon comes to the Sextile of the place she was in then. Hippocrates was against Astrologers, as appears by this Aphorism: And our College, the Physicians, hug his writing under their arms but follow him as much as the Pope follows Saint Peter.

10. Note the place the moon is in at the Decumbiture; then view the sick body, when the moon comes to the Sextile of that place: If you find ill Symptoms of the sick body, then you may fear death, when she comes to the Quartile of that place, and you have cause enough.

11. Short Maladies are better judged of than long; a great deal of time may produce more alteration than a little.

12. If Fevers happen to women in childbed, begin the Calculation at the time of her delivery, and not at the Initiation of the sickness, and take their Crisis that way.

13. If the Fever continues to the third Crisis, which is not often; you may presage bleeding at the Nose; and it is twenty to one, it comes not upon the day of the third Crisis, or near it.

14. If the Patient bleed not at the Nose, be sure he has an Apostume in some of the inferior parts of his body.

15. Flux of blood in such a case most usually happens to people that are under thirty years of age; apostumes to them that are older.

16. If the sick find a vehement pain about his forehead, or places near it; he is very subject to bleed at the Nose, and that may save his life.

17. Young persons oftener die at the first Crisis in Fevers, than ancient; and the reason is because their nature is hotter, and the more subject to take fire; for he that knows but his A. B. C.'s in Physic, knows a Fever comes of heat.

18. Old persons sooner die upon relapses than young; and the reason is because their bodies are weaker.

19. Ulcerations in the throat are usually mortal in hot diseases.

20. Fevers continue longer in ancient people than they do in young; and the reason is because the bodies of ancient people are colder; dry wood will burn most violently it is confessed: but wet wood will be longer a burning.

21. Ancient people are more subject to quartan Agues than young; and the reason is because Saturn causes them: a child will leave playing with his Father, to play with its equals.

Presages of the Quinsy.

1. All Quinsies are extreme dangerous, and sometimes mortal.

2. The most dangerous signs in a Quinsy are great pain, great difficulty in breathing, yet no swelling outwardly appearing; for if the swelling appears, the external part of the throat is most afflicted. And if you do not believe better to have the External part of the throat afflicted than the Internal; I wish you did.

3. Here you find that in the Quinsy, it is better when they appear outwardly, than when they do not.

4. If the swelling appears not outwardly, they usually kill within four days at the furthest, although no Crisis comes at that time. My own opinion is, though I hold an absolute truth in the Crisis, as I have laid them down in this book: yet withal, I know as well, that there is a difference to be made between the time that the disease overcomes the vitals, and the time of the dissolution; as also that in a proper acute disease.

5. The moon to the semi Sextile of the place she was in at the Decumbiture, often kills; because she is then in a sign opposite in respect of nature, sex, and time.

6. If a red tumor appears outwardly, and falls in again, the danger of death is great. Life may borrow a little time, and so forth, but 'tis to be feared, must be forced to yield to her enemy Death at last.

7. If the tumor in a Quinsy increase upon a Critical day, and break neither inwardly nor outwardly, death or a relapse, or something as bad is to be feared, though the Patient feels case for the time.

Presages by the Uvula.

The presages are but few; happily honest Hippocrates whom Authors call divine for his ingenuity rather than his religion, because the diseases in this part of the body are but few, and those few appear but seldom.

1. Incision in the Uvula, Gargarion, or Columella, when it is swollen, red, or gross, is dangerous; Physicians love to trouble your pates with hard words; for if they would write plain English, they could not make silly people believe wonders, and then their Diana would down; you shall find an explanation of all such words, which he that can but read his Primer shall find at the latter end of the book.

2. If the Uvula looks pale or livid, and the upper part not swelled, you may make an incision without danger.

3. Be sure you purge the belly before you be too busy in making incisions in those parts; thus Hippocrates.

The truth is, I cannot find any reason why any incision at all should be made there; a man may as well plead Excise as Custom for ought I know.

If there be an inflammation there, bloodletting in the arm will serve the turn; if putrefaction or ulcer, as sometimes, happen to such, as our company of Chirurgeons Flux for the French pox, either for want of care or skill, or something else; cleansing medicines will do the deed. I do not in this Treatise profess to write an Anatomy; if I did I could tell you what the use of the Uvula was, and how difficult an incision there is, and how dangerous the effects of it may prove; but I pass it and come to,

Presages of Vomiting in fevers.

1. First of all when there appears black things, or things like flies, before the eyes of him that has a

fever, viz. when he thinks he sees flies, when there's no such thing near him; be sure the sick will vomit yellow choler, and the surer if withal he find an illness at his stomach.

2. If there be a stiffness and chilliness in those parts near the Hypochondria, the vomiting will the sooner be hastened.

3. My Author does not tell whether this vomiting be good or bad in a fever; therefore, I'll tell it you for him; it shows strength of nature; therefore, take it as a hopeful sign; the choler which is vomited up lies in the stomach; and that's not the place dame nature has provided to hold choler. Dame nature is like a Prince in the body, and holds in tenure by Soccage, under Almighty God; and if she can expel her enemy out of her dominions, does she not do well?

4. If together with what was mentioned before, there happen swelling or ringings, by reason of wind under one of the sides, be not too hasty to predict vomiting; it is more probable to be only bleeding at the nose.

5. Bleeding at the nose in such a case usually happens to people under 30 years of age, vomiting to such as are older.

6. These presages has Hippocrates left to posterity verified by his own experience; I have ordered them for your own good, as well as I can; I have given you the reasons of some of them; because I would instruct you; of others I have not, because I would encourage you to study; for take this for an absolute truth, my writings may teach you, but it is your selves must make yourselves Physicians; Doctor Reason told me these presages were true. And Experience tells you by my pen, that you shall find them so. I now take my leave of you for this

time, and withal tell you, that if you be not so free
to do good to others, as I am to you, look to answer
for it another day at the general account.

I remain Yours to do you good whilst I remain amongst
the Living. Nich. Culpepper.

15 Aprilis 1651. Imprimatur, JOHN BOOKER.

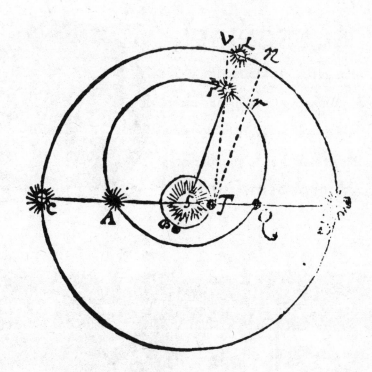

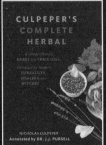
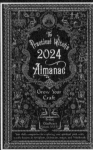
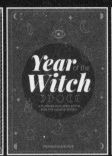
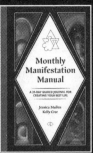
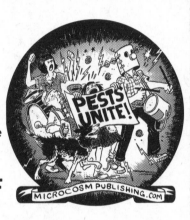
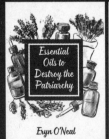
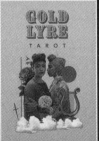
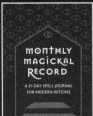
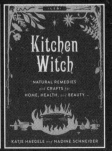